A

A (accommodation)
AA (amplitude of accommodation)
AACG (acute angle closure glaucoma)
ab externo incision
abducens (VI) nerve
abducens paralysis
abducens-facial paralysis
abduction
abductor muscles
aberrant regeneration
aberration
ablepharia
ablepharon
ablepharous
ablephary
ablepsia
ablepsy
abrasio
    a. corneae
abrasion
    corneal a.
abrin
abscess
    corneal a.
    lacrimal a.
    orbital a.
    ring a.
abscessus
    a. siccus corneae
abscission
    corneal a.
absinthe
absolute accommodation
absolute glaucoma
absolute hemianopia
absolute hyperopia
absolute scotoma
absolute strabismus
absorptive lenses
abstraction
AC (anterior chamber)
AC/A ratio (accommodative convergence/accommodation ratio)
Acc (accommodation)
accessory fibers
accessory nucleus
accessory organs of eye
accidental image
accommodation
    absolute a.
    binocular a.
    excessive a.
    negative a.
    positive a.
    relative a.
    subnormal a.
accommodation iridoplegia
accommodation reflex
accommodative

Additional Entries

_____
_____
_____
_____
_____

accommodative asthenopia
accommodative convergence
accommodative cyclophoria
accommodative esotropia
accommodative palsy
accommodative spasm
accommodative strabismus
accommodative target
accommodometer
Accugel (contact lenses, soft)
Accugel Thin (contact lenses, soft)
acetazolamide
acetylcholine chloride
ACG (angle closure glaucoma)
achloropsia
achlys
achromat
achromatic lens
achromatic perimetry
achromatic threshold
achromatic vision
achromatopia
achromatopic
achromatopsia
Achromycin
acid
    boric a.
    hyaluronic a.
    mucoitin-sulfuric a.
    perosmic a.
acinesia
acne rosacea keratitis
acorea
acoustic spots
acquired astigmatism
acquired esotropia
acritochromacy

acrochordon
acrylic lens implant
A.C.S. Alcon closure system
A.C.S. needle
actinic conjunctivitis
actinic keratitis
actinic retinitis
acuity
acute angle closure glaucoma
acute congestive glaucoma
acute contagious conjunctivitis
Adams operation
adaptation
    color a.
    dark a.
    light a.
    photopic a.
    retinal a.
adaptometer
    color a.
adduction
adduction muscles
adherent cataract
Adie's pupil
Adie's syndrome
adipose body of orbit
Adler operation
adnexa
    a. oculi
adolescent cataract
Adsorbocarpine
Adsorbonac
Adsorbotear
advancement
Aebli corneal scissors
aerosol keratitis
afferent defect
afferent nerve

Additional Entries
_____
_____
_____
_____

after-cataract
afterimage
aftervision
Agamodistomum
    A. ophthalmobium
aglaucopsia
aglaukopsia
Agnew operation
agnosia
    visual a.
agonist
Agrikola retractor
AHM (anterior hyaloid membrane)
air-block glaucoma
AIRLens contact lens (Wesley-Jessen)
air-puff tonometer
Akarpine
Ak-Chlor
Ak-Cide
Ak-Con
Ak-Con-A
Ak-Dex
Ak-Dilate
Ak-Fluor
akinesia
    O'Brien a.
    Van Lint a.
Ak-Mycin
Ak-NaCl
Ak-Nefrin
aknephascopia
Akorn balanced salt solution
Ak-Pentolate
Ak-Poly-Bac
Ak-Pred
Ak-Spore
Ak-Spore H.C.
Ak-Sulf
Ak-Taine
Ak-Tate
Ak-Trol
Akwa Tears
ala
    a. minor ossis sphenoidalis
Albalon
Albalon-A
albinism
    ocular a.
albinoidism
albinotic fundus
albuginea
    a. oculi
albugo
Alcaine
Alcmaeon of Crotona
Alcon cryophake
Alcon hand cautery
Alcon I-knife
Alcon Laboratories
Alcon Microsponge
Alcon surgical knife
Alexander's law
alexia
    optical a.
    subcortical a.
alexic
Ali ben Iza
Alidase
alkaptonuria
Allen operation
Allen-Braley implant
Allergan Humphrey
Allergan Humphrey laser
Allergan Humphrey lensometer

Additional Entries

Allergan Humphrey perimeter
Allergan Humphrey refractor
Allergan lensometer
Allergan Medical Optics
Allergan Medical Optics photokeratoscope
Allergan Pharmaceuticals
allergic conjunctivitis
allergic pannus
allokeratoplasty
allophthalmia
Allport operation
Almocarpine
alphabet keratitis
Alpha Chymar
alpha chymotrypsin
Alport's syndrome
Alsus-Knapp operation
alternate cover test
alternate day esotropia
alternating esotropia
alternating mydriasis
alternating strabismus
alternating sursumduction
alternating tropia
altitudinal hemianopia
Alvis operation
Alza Corporation
amacrine cells
amasthenic
amaurosis
    albuminuric a.
    Burns's a.
    cat's eye a.
    central a.
    cerebral a.
    congenital a.
    diabetic a.

amaurosis *(continued)*
    fugax, a.
    hysteric a.
    intoxication a.
    Leber's congenital a.
    reflex a.
    saburral a.
    uremic a.
amaurotic
amaurotic nystagmus
amaurotic pupil
ambiopia
amblyope
amblyopia
    alcoholica, a.
    ametropic a.
    arsenic a.
    color a.
    crapulosa, a.
    crossed a.
    cruciata, a.
    deprivation a.
    ex anopsia, a.
    functional a.
    hysteric a.
    nocturnal a.
    of arrest, a.
    of disuse, a.
    postmarital a.
    quinine a.
    reflex a.
    refractive a.
    strabismic a.
    suppression a.
    tobacco a.
    toxic a.
    traumatic a.
    uremic a.

Additional Entries

amblyopiatrics
amblyoscope
American Hydron
American IOL International lens
American Medical Optics intraocular lens
American Optical photocoagulator
ametropia
    axial a.
    curvature a.
    index a.
    position a.
    refractive a.
ametropic
Ammon operation
Ammon's scleral prominence
amnesic color blindness
AMO intraocular lens (Allergan Medical Optics)
amotio
    a. retinae
AMPPE (acute multifocal placoid pigment epitheliopathy)
amphamphoterodiplopia
amphiblestritis
amphodiplopia
amphoterodiplopia
amplitude
    a. of accommodation
    a. of convergence
ampulla
    a. canaliculi lacrimalis
    a. ductus lacrimalis
    a. of lacrimal canaliculis
Amsler grid
Amsler operation
Amsof (contact lenses, soft)
Amsofthin (contact lenses, soft)
amyloidosis
anaclasimeter
anaclasis
anaclisis
anaglyph
anagnosasthenia
Anagnostakis (Hotz-Anagnostakis) operation
analgesia
    permeation a.
    surface a.
anangioid disk
anaphylactic conjunctivitis
anatomic equator
anatropia
anatropic
anesthesia
    retrobulbar a.
    topical a.
aneurysm
    miliary a.
    orbital a.
Angelucci operation
Angelucci syndrome
angioid streaks
angioscotoma
angioscotometry
angle
    alpha a.
    anamoly, a. of
    anterior chamber, a. of
    biorbital a.
    convergence, a. of
    deviation, a. of

Additional Entries

angle *(continued)*
    direction, a. of
    filtration a.
    gamma a.
    incidence, a. of
    iridial a.
    iridocorneal a.
    iris, a. of
    kappa a.
    lambda a.
    lateral a. of eye
    medial a. of eye
    minimum visual a.
    ocular a.
    ocularis, a. of
    optic a.
    refraction, a. of
    squint a.
    visual a.
angle-closure glaucoma
angle-recession glaucoma
angor
    a. ocularis
angular blepharitis
angular conjunctivitis
angular distance
angulus
    a. iridocornealis
    a. oculi lateralis
    a. oculi medialis
anianthinopsy
aniridia
aniseikonia
aniseikonic
anisoaccommodation
anisochromatic
anisocoria
anisometropia
anisometropic
anisophoria
anisopia
ankyloblepharon
    a. filiforme adnatum
    a. totale
annular corneal graft
annular scleritis
annular scotoma
annular staphyloma
annular synechia
annular ulcer
annulus
    a. ciliaris
    a. of Zinn
anomalopia
anomaloscope
anomalous retinal correspondence
anomalous trichromatism
anomaly, Axenfeld's
anophthalmia
anophthalmus
anopia
anopsia
anorthopia
anotropia
antagonist
    contralateral a.
    ipsilateral a.
antazoline phosphate ophthalmic solution
anterior axial developmental cataract
anterior chamber of eye
anterior choroiditis
anterior embryotoxon
anterior epithelium of cornea

Additional Entries

_____
_____
_____
_____
_____

anterior limiting lamina
anterior pole of eyeball
anterior pole of lens
anterior pyramidal cataract
anterior scleritis
anterior sclerotomy
anterior staphyloma
anterior symblepharon
anterior synechia
anterior uveitis
Anthony compressor
antigen
    lens a.
antihyaluronidase
antimetropia
antimongoloid slant
antixerophthalmic
antrophose
anulus
    a. iridis major
    a. iridis minor
    a. of conjunctiva
    a. tendineus communis
AO Reichert Scientific
   Instruments
Aosoft (contact lenses, soft)
A-pattern
aphacia
aphacic
aphakia
aphakic
aphakic glaucoma
aphasia
    optic a.
aphose
aphotesthesia
apical clearance
apical radius
apical zone
aplanatic focus
aplanatism
aplasia
    retinal a.
aponeurosis
aponeurosis of Zinn
apoplectic glaucoma
apoplectic retinitis
apotripsis
apparatus
    ciliary a.
    lacrimal a.
    suspensorius lentis, a.
appendage
    a's of the eye
applanation
applanation tonometer
applanation tonometry
applanometer
aqua
    a. oculi
Aquaflex
Aquaflex (contact lenses, soft)
Aquasight (contact lenses, soft)
aqueous
aqueous flare
aqueous humor
aqueous outflow
aqueous paracentesis
aqueous veins
aquocapsulitis
AR-1000 refractor
AR-1600 refractor
arachnoid sheath
arborescent cataract
ARC (abnormal retinal
   correspondence)

Additional Entries

arc
    a. of contact
arc-flash conjunctivitis
arc perimeter
arc scotoma
arch
    orbital a. of frontal bone
    superciliary a.
    supraorbital a. of frontal bone
arcus
    a. lipoides corneae
    a. palpebralis superior
    a. senilis
    a. superciliaris
areolar central choroiditis
areolar choroiditis
argamblyopia
argon laser
    Allergan Humphrey l.
    Biophysic Medical l.
    CILCO l.
    Coherent Medical l.
    CooperVision l.
    CooperVision Surgical l.
    SITE l.
Argyll Robertson operation
Argyll Robertson pupil
argyria
argyriasis
argyrism
argyrosis
ariboflavinosis
aridosiliculose cataract
aridosiliquate cataract
Arion operation
Arlt epicanthus repair
Arlt eyelid repair technique
Arlt loop
Arlt-Jaesche operation
Arlt-Jaesche recessus
Arlt-Jaesche sinus
Arlt-Jaesche trachoma
Arlt pterygium excision
arrachement
Arrowhead (Wicherkiewicz) operation
Arruga capsule forceps
Arruga cataract extraction
Arruga dacryostomy
Arruga encircling suture
Arruga implant
Arruga keratoplasty
Arruga retractor
Arruga tenotomy
Arruga-Berens operation
Arruga-Moura-Brazil orbital implant
arsenic amblyopia
arteriae
    a. cerebri
    a. cerebri anterior
    a. cerebri media
    a. ciliares anteriores
    a. ciliares posteriores breves
    a. ciliares posteriores longae
    a. conjunctivales anteriores
    a. conjunctivales posteriores
    a. episclerales
    a. hyaloidea
    a. lacrimalis
    a. ophthalmica
    a. palpebrales laterales

Additional Entries

arteriae *(continued)*
    a. palpebrales mediales
    a. supraorbitalis
    a. supratrochlearis
    a. temporalis superficialis
    a. zygomaticoorbitalis
arteriola
    a. macularis inferior
    a. macularis superior
    a. medialis retinae
    a. nasalis retinae inferior
    a. nasalis retinae superior
    a. temporalis retinae inferior
    a. temporalis retinae superior
arterial circle of iris, lesser
arterial circle of iris, greater
arteriole
    macular a., inferior
    macular a., superior
    medial a. of retina
    nasal a. of retina, inferior
    nasal a. of retina, superior
    temporal a. of retina, inferior
    temporal a. of retina, superior
arteritis
    temporal a.
artery
    central a. of retina
    ciliary a's, anterior
    ciliary a's, long
    ciliary a's, posterior, long
    ciliary a's, posterior, short
    ciliary a's, short

artery *(continued)*
    conjunctival a's, anterior
    conjunctival a's, posterior
    copper-wire a.
    cork-screw a.
    episcleral a.
    infraorbital a.
    ophthalmic a.
    supraorbital a.
    tarsal a., lateral
    tarsal a's, medial
    zygomaticoorbital a.
arthro-ophthalmopathy
    hereditary progressive a.
artificial pupil
artificial silk keratitis
A-scan
A-scan ultrasound
Ascher's glass-rod phenomenon
Ascher's syndrome
Aseptron II
aspheric lens implant
aspherical cornea
aspirator
    Nugent soft cataract a.
asteroid hyalitis
asteroid hyalosis
asthenic orthophoria
asthenopia
    accommodative a.
    muscular a.
    nervous a.
    retinal a.
asthenopic
astigmagraph
astigmatic
astigmatic clock
astigmatic dial

Additional Entries

astigmatism
    acquired a.
    against the rule, a.
    compound a.
    congenital a.
    corneal a.
    direct a.
    hypermetropic a.
    hyperopic a.
    hyperopic a., simple
    inverse a.
    irregular a.
    lenticular a.
    mixed a.
    myopic a.
    myopic a., compound
    myopic a., simple
    oblique a.
    physiological a.
    regular a.
    simple a.
    with the rule, a.
astigmatometer
astigmatoscope
astigmatoscopy
astigmia
astigmic
astigmometer
astigmometry
astigmoscope
ataxia
    ocular a.
atopic cataract
atopic conjunctivitis
atresia
    a. iridis
atretoblepharia
atretopsia

Atropair
atrophia
    a. bulbi
    a. bulborum hereditaria
    a. choroideae et retinae
    a. dolorosa
atrophic
atrophic excavation
atrophy
    Leber's optic a.
    optic a.
    optic a., primary
    optic a., secondary
    progressive choroidal a.
atropine
atropine conjunctivitis
atropine sulfate
atropine sulfate S.O.P.
attention reflex of pupil
audiovisual
audito-oculogyric reflex
Aureomycin
auricular glaucoma
autofundoscope
autofundoscopy
autokeratometer (Canon U.S.A.)
autokeratoplasty
automated hemisphere
    perimeter
automated refractor
auto-ophthalmoscope
auto-ophthalmoscopy
autophthalmoscope
Autoref keratometer RK-1
    (Canon U.S.A.)
autorefractor
auxiometer
auxometer

Additional Entries

_____
_____
_____
_____

Ax (axis of cylindric lens)
axanthopsia
Axenfeld loops
Axenfeld syndrome
axial ametropia
axial cataract
axial fusiform developmental cataract
axial hyperopia
axial length
axial myopia
axiliary cataract
axis
    bulbi externus, a.
    bulbi internus, a.
    external a. of eye
    Fick, a. of
    internal a. of eye
    lens, a. of

axis *(continued)*
    lentis, a.
    oculi externa, a.
    oculi interna, a.
    optic a.
    optical a.
    principal a.
    pupillary a.
    sagittal a. of eye
    sagittal a. of eye, secondary
    vertical a. of eye
    visual a.
axometer
axoneme
axonometer
Ayer forceps
Ayerst Epitrate
Ayerst Laboratories

Additional Entries

B

bacillary layer
Bacillus subtilis
bacitracin
back vertex power
bacterial conjunctivitis
Badal's operation
Bagolini lenses
Baird forceps
balanced salt solution
Balint's syndrome
Ballen-Alexander retractor
Ballet's sign
band
    zonular b.
band keratopathy
bandage
    binocle b.
    Borsch's b.
band-shaped keratitis
band-shaped keratopathy
Bangerter operation
bank keratitis
Banner snare
bar reader
Bard's sign
Bardelli operation
Bard-Parker knife
Barkan cyclodialysis
Barkan goniotomy
Barkan implant
Barkan-Cordes operation
Barnes-Hind
Barnes-Hind cleaning and
    soaking solution
Barnes-Hind soft contact lenses

Barraquer zonulolysis
Barraquer forceps
Barraquer keratomileusis
Barraquer implant
Barre's sign
barrel distortion
Barrie Jones operation
Barrier sheet
basal lamina of choroid
basal lamina of ciliary body
basal ophthalmoplegia
base-down prism
base-in prism
base-out prism
base-up prism
Basol-S
bathomorphic
Batten-Mayou disease
Baumgarten's gland
Bausch & Lomb
bay
    lacrimal b.
bear tracks
Beard knife
Beard-Cutler operation
Beaver blade
Beaver knife
bedewing
Beer's collyrium
Beer's knife
Beer's operation
Behr's disease
Behr's pupil
Bell erysiphake
Bell's palsy

Additional Entries

___
___
___
___
___

belonoskiascopy
Benedict operation
Benson's disease
Beraud's valve
Berens corneal knife
Berens lens expressor
Berens orbital implant
Berens pterygium transplant
Berens-Rosa scleral implant
Berens sclerectomy
Berens-Smith operation
Berger's sign (symptom)
Berke operation
Berke-Motais operation
Berlin's disease
Berlin's edema
Berman localizer
Bernheimer's fibers
Berry's circle
Best's disease
Betagan
Bethke iridectomy
Betoptic
BI (base in prism)
Bianchi's valve
b.i.d. (twice a day)
Bielschowsky head tilt test
Bielschowsky operation
Bielschowsky-Jansky disease
bifixation
bifocal
bifocal fixation
bifocal glasses
bifoveal fixation
bilateral hemianopia
bilateral strabismus
binasal hemianopia
Binkhorst collar stud lens implant

binocle bandage
binocular
binocular accommodation
binocular diplopia
binocular fixation
binocular fusion
binocular hemianopia
binocular indirect ophthalmoscopy
binocular ophthalmoscope
binocular parallax
binocular polyopia
binocular rivalry
binocular strabismus
binocular vision
binoculus
binophthalmoscope
binoscope
biomicroscope
   slit lamp b.
biomicroscopy
Bio-Optics
Bio-Optics camera
Bio-Optics clinical specular microscope
Bio-Pen hand-held biometric ruler (Intermedics Intraocular)
biophotometer
Biophysic Medical
Biophysic Medical laser
biorbital
biorbital angle
bipolar
   cone b.
   giant b.
   rod b.
bi-prism applanation tonometer (Reichert)

Additional Entries
_____
_____
_____
_____
_____

Birch-Hirschfeld operation
Birch-Hirschfeld lamp
Bishop-Harmon irrigator
Bi-Soft contact lenses, soft
bitemporal hemianopia
Bitot's spots
Bjerrum's scotoma
Bjerrum's scotometer
Bjerrum's screen
Bjerrum's sign
BKS-1000 Refractive Set
   (Allergan Medical Optics)
black cataract
black sunburst
blade
    Beaver b.
Blair operation
Blasius operation
Blaskovics operation
Blaskovics-Doyen
blear eye
bleb
blennorrhea
    adultorum, b.
    neonatorum, b.
    inclusion b.
blennorrheal conjunctivitis
Bleph-10
Blephamide
blepharadenitis
blepharal
blepharectomy
blepharelosis
blepharism
blepharitis
    angularis, b.
    ciliaris, b.
    marginalis, b.

blepharitis *(continued)*
   nonulcerative b.
   seborrheic b.
   squamous seborrheic b.
blepharoadenitis
blepharoadenoma
blepharoatheroma
blepharochalasis
blepharochromidrosis
blepharoclonus
blepharoconjunctivitis
blepharodiastasis
blepharoncus
blepharopachynsis
blepharophimosis
blepharoplasty
blepharoplegia
blepharoptosis
blepharopyorrhea
blepharorrhaphy
blepharospasm
    essential b.
    symptomatic b.
blepharosphincterectomy
blepharostat
blepharostenosis
blepharosynechia
blepharotomy
blepharoxysis
Blessig's groove
blind
blind spot
blindness
    amnesic color b.
    blue b.
    blue-yellow b.
    Bright's b.
    color b.

Additional Entries

blindness *(continued)*
    concussion b.
    cortical b.
    cortical psychic b.
    day b.
    eclipse b.
    epidemic b.
    flash b.
    flight b.
    functional b.
    green b.
    legal b.
    letter b.
    mind b.
    moon b.
    night b.
    note b.
    object b.
    psychic b.
    red b.
    red-green b.
    river b.
    snow b.
    soul b.
    syllabic b.
    text b.
    total b.
    twilight b.
    word b.
Blink-N-Clean
blink reflex
Blinx
blood cataract
blow-out fracture
blown pupil
blue blindness
blue cataract
blue dot cataract
blue sclera
blue spot
blue-yellow blindness
blur and clear
blur point
B-mode handpiece
BO (base out prism)
bobbing
Boberg-Ans lens implant
Bochdalek's valve
bodies, Elschnig's (pearls)
body
    adipose b. of orbit
    ciliary b.
    Elschnig b.
    Landolt's b.
    lenticular b.
    Lipschutz b.
    nigroid b.
    trachoma b.
    vitreous b.
Bohm's operation
Boil-n-Soak
Bonaccolto monoplex orbital
    implant
Bonaccolto ring
Bonaccolto-Flieringa scleral
    ring
Bonaccolto-Flieringa operation
Bonn forceps
Bonnett operation
Bonnier's syndrome
Bonzel's operation
border
    orbital b. of sphenoid bone
boric acid
Borsch's bandage
Borthen operation

Additional Entries

Bossalino blepharoplasty
bottlemaker's cataract
Botvin forceps
bounding mydriasis
bounding pupil
bouquet of Rochon-Duvigneaud
Bowman cataract needle
Bowman's lamina
Bowman's layer
Bowman's membrane
Bowman's muscle
Bowman's tubes
boxcarring
Bozzi's foramen
brachium
    conjunctival b., anterior
    conjunctival b., posterior
brachymetropia
brachymetropic
Bracken forceps
Braid effect
Braid's strabismus
Brailey's operation
Brawner orbital implant
brawny scleritis
breakup time
Brickner's sign
bridge coloboma
Bridge operation
Briggs operation
Bright's blindness
Bright's disease
Bright's eye
Brodmann area 8
Brodmann area 17
Brodmann area 18
Brodmann area 19
Bromley operation

Bronson operation
Bronson-Turz retractor
brown cataract
Brown-Dohlman corneal
    implant
Brown-Pusey trephine
Bruch's gland
Bruch's membrane
Bruchner test
Brucke's muscle
brunescent cataract
brush
    Haidinger's b.
Brushfield's spots
Brushfield-Wyatt syndrome
B-Scan ultrasound
BSS
BSS Plus
BSV (binocular single vision)
BU (base up prism)
buckle
Budinger blepharoplasty
Buettner-Parel vitreous cutter
bufilcon A
bulb
    b. of eye
bulbar conjunctiva
bulbocapnine
bulbus
bulbus oculi
bullous keratopathy
bull's-eye retinopathy
bullular canal
Bumke's pupil
Bunge's spoon
buphthalmia
buphthalmos
Burch operation

Additional Entries

_____
_____
_____
_____
_____

Burn's amaurosis
Burow operation
Burroughs Wellcome
Busacca nodules
BUT (breakup time)

Buzzi's operation
BVA (best corrected visual acuity)
b-wave
Byron Smith operation

Additional Entries

C

C (cylindric lens or cylinder)
Cairns trabeculectomy
calcareous cataract
calcareous conjunctivitis
calcarine fissure
Caldwell-Luc operation
Calhoun-Hagler operation
caliculus
    c. ophthalmicus
caligo
    c. corneae
    c. lentis
    c. pupillae
caliper
Callahan operation
Calmette's ophthalmoreaction
caloric nystagmus
caloric testing
camera
    anterior bulbi, c.
    Bio-Optics c.
    Canon U.S.A. c.
    Carl Zeiss c.
    Coburn c.
    CooperVision Diagnostic Imaging c.
    CooperVision PRO-CMC 200 color video c.
    fundus/retinal c.
    GRC-WT fundus c.
    Keeler c.
    Kowa hand c.
    Kowa Optimed c.
    Kowa RC-2 fundus c.
    Nikon external c.

camera *(continued)*
    oculi, c.
    oculi anterior, c.
    oculi posterior, c.
    ophthalmoscope c.
    posterior bulbi, c.
    PRO-CMC 200 color video c.
    Reichert c.
    Schepens binocular indirect c.
    Topcon c.
Campbell retractor
campimeter
Campodonico operation
canal
    bullular c.
    central c. of vitreous
    ethmoid c., anterior
    Ferrein's c.
    Hannover's c.
    infraorbital c.
    lacrimal c.
    nasal c.
    nasolacrimal c.
    optic c.
    orbital c.
    orbital c., anterior internal
    orbital c., posterior internal
    ruffed c.
    Schlemm's c.
    scleral c.
    scleroticochoroidal c.
    Sondermann's c.
    supraciliary c.

Additional Entries

canal *(continued)*
    supraoptic c.
    supraorbital c.
    tarsal c.
canalicular
canalicular duct
canaliculi
canaliculitis
canaliculization
canaliculodacryocystostomy
canaliculorhinostomy
canaliculus
    c. lacrimalis
canalis
    c. infraorbitalis
    c. opticus
candlewax dripping
cannula
    Gass c.
Canon auto acuitometer (Canon U.S.A.)
Canon U.S.A.
Canon U.S.A. camera
Canon U.S.A. perimeter
Canon U.S.A. refractor
Cantelli's sign
canthectomy
canthi
canthitis
cantholysis
canthoplasty
canthotomy
canthus
capsular cataract
capsular glaucoma
capsule
    c. of lens
capsulectomy

capsulorhexis

capsulitis
capsulolenticular
capsulolenticular cataract
capsulotome
capsulotomy
carbachol ophthalmic solution
cardinal points
Cardona focalizing fundus lens implant
Cardona gonio-focalizing lens implant
Carl Zeiss, Inc.
Carl Zeiss camera
Carl Zeiss laser
Carl Zeiss lensometer
Carl Zeiss refractor
Carter sphere introducer
Carter's operation
cartilage
    central c.
    ciliary c.
    palpebral c.
caruncula
    c. lacrimalis
Casanellas operation
case
    trial c.
Casey's operation
Caspar's ring
Castroviejo keratoplasty
Castroviejo needle holder
Castroviejo orbital implant
Castroviejo scissors
Castroviejo suture forceps
Castroviejo-Arruga forceps
Castroviejo-Kalt needle holder
Castroviejo-Scheie cyclodiathermy

Additional Entries

cat's eye amaurosis
cat's eye pupil
cat's eye syndrome
cataphoria
cataract
    adherent c.
    adolescent c.
    after c.
    anterior axial c.
    anterior pyramidal c.
    arborescent c.
    aridosiliculose c.
    aridosiliquate c.
    atopic c.
    axial c.
    axial fusiform c.
    axiliary c.
    black c.
    blue c.
    blue dot c.
    bottlemaker's c.
    brown c.
    brunescent c.
    calcareous c.
    capsular c.
    capsulolenticular c.
    central c.
    cerulean c.
    choroidal c.
    complete c.
    complete congenital c.
    complicated c.
    congenital c.
    contusion c.
    coralliform c.
    coronary c.
    coronary of Vogt c.
    cortical c.

cataract *(continued)*
    cupuliform c.
    cystic c.
    degenerative c.
    developmental c.
    diabetic c.
    dry-shelled c.
    electric c.
    embryonal nuclear c.
    fibroid c.
    floriform c.
    fluid c.
    fusiform c.
    general c.
    glassblower's c.
    glaucomatous c.
    gray c.
    green c.
    hard c.
    heat c.
    heat-ray c.
    hedger's heterochromic c.
    hypermature c.
    immature c.
    incipient c.
    infantile c.
    intumescent c.
    irradiation c.
    juvenile c.
    lacteal c.
    lamellar c.
    lenticular c.
    lightning c.
    mature c.
    membranous c.
    milky c.
    mixed c.
    morgagnian c.

Additional Entries

cataract *(continued)*
- naphthalinic c.
- nuclear c.
- overripe c.
- partial c.
- perinuclear c.
- peripheral c.
- poisoning c.
- polar c., anterior
- polar c., posterior
- primary c.
- progressive c.
- puddler's c.
- punctuate c.
- pyramidal c.
- radiation c.
- reduplication c.
- ripe c.
- sanguineous c.
- secondary c.
- sedimentary c.
- senile c.
- senile cortical c.
- senile nuclear c.
- siliculose c.
- siliquose c.
- snowflake c.
- snowstorm c.
- Soemmering's ring c.
- soft c.
- spear c.
- spindle c.
- stationary c.
- stellate c.
- subcapsular c.
- sunflower c.
- sutural c.
- total c.

cataract *(continued)*
- toxic c.
- traumatic c.
- tremulous c.
- zonular c.

cataract gonfle operation
cataract secondary to disease
cataracta
- c. accreta
- c. brunescens
- c. cerulea
- c. congenita membranacea
- c. coronaria
- c. membranacea accreta
- c. neurodermatica
- c. nigra
- c. ossea
- c. syndermotica

cataractogenic
cataractopiesis
cataractous
Catarase
catarrh
- spring c.
- vernal c.

catarrhal conjunctivitis
catarrhal corneal ulcer
catheterization of the lacrimonasal duct
cautery
- Alcon hand c.
- Parker-Heath c.
- Todd c.

cavern
- Schnabel's c.

Cavitron-Kelman cataract surgical system unit

Additional Entries

Cavitron-Kelman KCP
  phacoemulsifier aspirator
Cavitron/Kelman
  phacoemulsifier aspirator,
  Model 8001,
  (CooperVision Surgical)
Cavitron/Kelman
  phacoemulsifier aspirator,
  Model 9001,
  (CooperVision Surgical)
cc (with correction)
CE-82 cryosurgical system
  (Frigitronics)
cecal
cell
  bipolar retinal c.
  corneal c.
  visual c.
  wing c.
cell and flare
cellulitis
  orbital c.
Celsus operation
Celsus-Hotz operation
center
  optic c.
  rotation, c. of
centrage
central amaurosis
central angiospastic retinitis
central artery of retina
central canal of vitreous
central cataract
central choroiditis
central developmental cataract
central disk-shaped retinopathy
central fixation
central fovea of retina
central fusion
central iridectomy
central scotoma
central serous retinopathy
central suppression
central vision
central visual acuity
centrally fixing eye
centraphose
centrocecal scotoma
cephalo-orbital index
ceratonosus
cerclage
cerebral amaurosis
cerebral phycomycosis
cerebral stratum of retinae
cerulean cataract
cerulean developmental cataract
Cetamide
Cetapred
CF (counting fingers)
CF/2 ft (counts fingers at 2 ft)
CF-60 U fundus camera (Canon
  U.S.A.)
chalazion
chalcosis
  c. corneae
  c. lentis
chalkitis
chamber
  anterior c. of eye
  aqueous c.
  vitreous c.
Chandler forceps
Chandler iridectomy
Chandler-Verhoeff lens
  extraction
Charcot's triad

Additional Entries

Charlin's syndrome
chart
    Guibor's c.
    reading c.
    Reuss' color c.
    Snellen's c.
check ligament
cheiroscope
chemical conjunctivitis
chemosis
cherry-red spot
chiasm
    optic c.
chiasma
    c. opticum
chiasma syndrome
chiasmatic syndrome
chiastometer
chief fibers
Chievitz layer
Chlorofair
chlorolabe
Chloromycetin
chlorophane
Chloroptic
chocked reflex
choke
    ophthalmovascular c.
choked disk
chondrogen
choriopapillaris
chorioretinal
chorioretinitis
chorioretinopathy
choroid
choroid fissure
choroidal
choroidal cataract
choroidal detachment
choroidal flush
choroidal hyperfluorescence
choroidal nevus
choroideremia
choroiditis
    anterior c.
    areolar c.
    areolar central c.
    diffuse c.
    disseminated c.
    Doyne's familial
        honeycombed c.
    exudative c.
    Forster's c.
    guttata senilis, c.
    metastatic c.
    senile macular exudative c.
    serosa, c.
    suppurative c.
    Tay's c.
choroidocyclitis
choroidoiritis
choroidopathy
choroidoretinitis
Choyce lens implant
chromatelopsia
chromatic aberration
chromatic dispersion
chromatic perimetry
chromatic vision
chromatodysopia
chromatometer
chromatopseudopsis
chromatopsia
chromatoptometer
chromatoptometry
chromatoskiameter

Additional Entries

chromic myopia
chromophobe adenoma
chromoretinography
chromoscope
chromoscopy
chronic narrow-angle glaucoma
chronic simple glaucoma
Ciaccio glands
Cibasoft
Cibasoft low plus
Cibasoft minus
Cibathin
Cibis liquid silicone procedure
cibisotome
cicatricial ectropion
cicatricial entropion
cicatricial strabismus
cicatrix
    filtering c.
CILCO corneascope
CILCO intraocular lens
CILCO laser
CILCO pachymeter (CooperVision Refractive Surgery)
CILCO perimeter
cilia
ciliaris
ciliariscope
ciliarotomy
ciliary
ciliary apparatus
ciliary arteries, anterior
ciliary arteries, long
ciliary arteries, posterior, short
ciliary arteries, short
ciliary body
ciliary body band

ciliary disk
ciliary folds
ciliary glands
ciliary glands of conjunctiva
ciliary margin of iris
ciliary muscle
ciliary nerves, long
ciliary nerves, short
ciliary processes
ciliary reflex
ciliary ring of iris
ciliary staphyloma
ciliary zonule
ciliate
ciliated
ciliectomy
cilioequatorial fibers
ciliogenesis
cilioretinal
cilioposterocapsular fibers
cilioscleral
ciliospinal
ciliospinal reflex
ciliotomy
cilium
cillosis
cinch
cinema eye
circadian heterotropia
circinate retinopathy
circle
    arterial c. of iris, greater
    arterial c. of iris, lesser
    arterial c. of Willis
    Berry's c.
    diffusion c.
    dispersion, c. of
    dissipation, c. of

Additional Entries

circle *(continued)*
    Haller, c. of
    Hovius, c. of
    iris, greater c. of
    iris, lesser c. of
    least confusion, c. of
    Minsky's c.
    vascular c. of optic nerve
    Zinn, c. of
circular fibers of ciliary muscle
circular synechia
circulus
    c. arteriosus halleri
    c. arteriosus iridis major
    c. arteriosus iridis minor
    c. vasculosus nervi optici
    c. zinnii
circumbulbar
circumcorneal
circumcorneal injection
circumduction
circumlental
circumlental space
circumocular
circumorbital
cirsophthalmia
cis retinal
cisterna
    c. chiasmatica
Citelli forceps
CK-1000 keratometer (Topcon Instrument)
CL-1500 lensmeter (Topcon Instrument)
Clark eye speculum
Clean-N-Soak
Clean-N-Soakit
Clean-N-Stow
Clear Eyes
Cleasby operation
cleft
    corneal c.
Clens
Clerz
Clerz 2
clinical specular microscope (Bio-Optics)
clock dial
C-loop single piece posterior chamber lens
Cloquet's canal
closed-angle glaucoma
CME (cystoid macular edema)
CMI (cytomegalic inclusion disease)
COAG (chronic open-angle glaucoma)
coagulator
    Mentor wet field c.
coarctate retina
Coat's retinitis
Coat's white ring
cobblestones
Coburn camera
Coburn I & A System (Coburn Optical)
Coburn I & A/vitrectomy (Coburn Optical)
Coburn IOL (Coburn Optical)
Coburn lensometer
Coburn Optical Industries
Coburn/Rayner intraocular lens
Coburn refractor
cochleopapillary reflex
Cogan-Boberg-Ans lens implant
Cogan's apraxia

Additional Entries

cogwheeling
Coherent 930 argon laser
 (Coherent Medical)
Coherent Medical
Coherent Medical 7910 Nd:YAG
 laser (Coherent Medical)
Coherent Medical 920 laser
 series (Coherent Medical)
Colesiota conjunctivae
Colettsia pecoris
Colibri forceps
collarette
colliculus
    c. superior laminae tecti
collodion dressing
collyrium
    Beer's c.
coloboma
    bridge c.
    choroid, c. of
    Fuch's c.
    iridis, c.
    iris, c. of
    lentis, c.
    lobuli, c.
    optic nerve, c. of
    palpebrale, c.
    retina, c. of
    retinae, c.
    typical c.
    vitreous, c. of
color
    confusion c.
    contrast c.
    incidental c.
    metameric c.
    pseudoisochromatic c.
color adaptation

color adaptometer
color amblyopia
color blindness
color deviant
color perimetry
color vision
columnar layer
coma aberration
Comberg operation
Combiline instrument system
Comfort
Comfort Drops
Comfort Tears
comitant heterotropia
comitant strabismus
commissura
    c. palpebrarum lateralis
    c. palpebrarum medialis
commissurae
commissure
    lateral c. of eyelids
    medial c. of eyelids
    supraoptic c.
commotio
    c. retinae
comparison eyepiece
compensating eyepiece
complementary after-image
complete cataract
complete congenital anterior
 polar developmental cataract
complete congenital posterior
 polar developmental cataract
complete hemianopia
complete iridoplegia
complicated cataract
complicated degenerative
 cataract

Additional Entries

compound astigmatism
compound eye
compound spectacles
compressor
    Anthony c.
concave lens
conclination
concomitant heterotropia
concomitant strabismus
concussion blindness
cone
    ocular c.
    retinal c.
    twin c.
    visual c.
cone fibers
cone granule
cone monochromacy
conformer
    Universal c.
confrontation fields
confusion
confusion color
congenital abducens-facial paralysis
congenital amaurosis
congenital astigmatism
congenital cataract
congenital glaucoma
congenital nystagmus
congenital pterygium
congestive glaucoma
congruous
congruous hemianopia
conical cornea
conjugate deviation
conjugate focus
conjugate movement
conjugate paralysis
conjugate point
conjunctiva
    bulbar c.
    palpebral c.
conjunctival
conjunctival arteries, anterior
conjunctival arteries, posterior
conjunctival brachium, posterior
conjunctival fold
conjunctival glands
conjunctival reaction
conjunctival reflex
conjunctival ring
conjunctival sac
conjunctival scraping
conjunctival veins
conjunctival xerosis
conjunctiviplasty
conjunctivitis
    actinic c.
    acute contagious c.
    allergic c.
    anaphylactic c.
    angular c.
    arc-flash c.
    atopic c.
    atropine c.
    blennorrheal c.
    calcareous c.
    catarrhal c.
    chemical c.
    croupous c.
    diphtheritic c.
    diplobacillary c.
    eczematous c.
    Egyptian c.
    epidemic c.

Additional Entries

conjunctivitis *(continued)*
    follicular c.
    gonococcal c.
    gonorrheal c.
    inclusion c.
    granular c.
    larval c.
    medicamentosa, c.
    membranous c.
    meningococcus c.
    molluscum c.
    Morax-Axenfeld's c.
    necroticans infectiosus, c.
    nodular c.
    Parinaud's c.
    Pascheff's c.
    phlyctenular c.
    prairie c.
    pseudomembranous c.
    purulent c.
    scrofular c.
    shipyard c.
    spring c.
    squirrel plague c.
    swimming pool c.
    trachomatous c.
    tularemic c.
    tularensis, c.
    uratic c.
    vernal c.
    welder's c.
    Widmark's c.
conjunctivodacryocystostomy
conjunctivoma
conjunctivoplasty
conjunctivorhinostomy
conoid
    Sturm's c.

conoid *(continued)*
    conomyoidin
    conophthalmus
    Conrad operation
    consensual
    consensual light reflex
    consensual reflex
    constant monocular tropia
    constant strabismus
    contact arc
    contact glasses
    contact lens (also see "lens")
    Contact Lens Technology
    contactogauge
    contactology
    contactoscope
    Contemporary Surgical Systems
    continuous fibers
    Contique
    contralateral
    contralateral antagonist
    contralateral synergist
    contrast
        high c.
        long-scale c.
        low c.
        short-scale c.
    contrast color
    contusion cataract
    conus
        distraction c.
        myopic c.
        optic disc, c. of
        supertraction c.
    converge
    convergence
        accommodative c.
        far point of c.

Additional Entries

convergence *(continued)*
   fusional c.
   near point of c.
   negative c.
   positive c.
   proximal c.
   relative c.
   tonic c.
   voluntary c.
convergence amplitudes
convergence-divergence
convergence insufficiency
convergence spasm
convergency reflex
convergent
convergent deviation
convergent ray
convergent strabismus
converging lens
convergiometer
convex lens
convexo-concave lens
Cooper (Reese-Jones) operation
CooperVision Diagnostic Imaging
CooperVision Diagnostic Imaging camera
CooperVision Diagnostic Imaging perimeter
CooperVision Diagnostic Imaging refractor
CooperVision IOL
CooperVision laser
CooperVision/Lasertek (laser system)
CooperVision Model 2000 Nd:YAG (CooperVision Laser)
CooperVision Model 2300 Nd:YAG (CooperVision Laser)
CooperVision Model 2500 Nd:YAG (CooperVision Laser)
CooperVision Model 40A argon (CooperVision Laser)
CooperVision Model 41K argon/krypton (CooperVision Laser)
CooperVision Model 7500 argon (CooperVision Laser)
CooperVision Model 8500 ACAP (CooperVision Surgical)
CooperVision Model 8500 argon/krypton (CooperVision Laser)
CooperVision/Moller microscope (CooperVision Surgical)
CooperVision Ophthalmic Products
CooperVision PRO-CMC 200 color video camera
CooperVision Refractive Surgery pachymeter (CooperVision Surgical)
CooperVision Refractive Surgery photokeratoscope
CooperVision Surgical laser
CooperVision System VI (CooperVision Surgical)
CooperVision System VI ultrasonic module (CooperVision Surgical)
Copeland Intralenses intraocular lens

Additional Entries

copper-wire arteries
copper-wire reflex
coralliform cataract
coralliform developmental cataract
coreclisis
corectasis
corectome
corectomedialysis
corectomy
corectopia
coredialysis
corediastasis
corelysis
coremorphosis
corenclisis
coreometer
coreometry
coreoplasty
corestenoma
    c. congenitum
coretomedialysis
coretomy
cork-screw arteries
cornea
    conical c.
    flat c.
    farinata, c.
    globosa, c.
    guttata, c.
    opaca, c.
    plana, c.
    verticillata, c.
    sugar-loaf c.
corneal
corneal abrasion
corneal abscess
corneal astigmatism
corneal bedewing
corneal button
corneal cap
corneal cleft
corneal dellen
corneal dystrophy
corneal edema
corneal endothelium
corneal epithelium
corneal fissure
corneal graft
    full-thickness c. g.
    lamellar c. g.
    mushroom c. g.
    penetrating c. g.
corneal microscope
corneal reflex
corneal staining test
corneal staphyloma
corneal tubes
corneal ulceration
corneal vascularization
corneal xerosis
corneitis
corneoblepharon
corneoiritis
corneomandibular reflex
corneomental reflex
corneopterygoid reflex
corneosclera
corneoscleral
cornpicker's pupil
corona
    ciliaris, c.
    Zinn's c.
coronary of Vogt developmental cataract
coroparelcysis

Additional Entries

coroplasty
coroscopy
corotomy
corpus
    c. ciliare
    c. ciliaris
correspondence
    anomalous retinal c.
    harmonious retinal c.
    retinal c.
corresponding points
cortex
cortical blindness
cortical cataract
cortical psychic blindness
cortical substance of lens
corticonuclear fibers
cortisone acetate ophthalmic suspension
Cortisporin
Corynebacterium
    C. xerose
    C. xerosis
cotton wool spots
couching
counts fingers
CPC (central posterior curve)
CPEO (chronic progressive external ophthalmoplegia)
CRA (central retinal artery)
CRAO (central retinal artery occlusion)
CR3-45NM non-mydriatic retinal camera (Canon U.S.A.)
craniofacial dysostosis
craniopharyngioma
Crawford operation
Crede's method
Crede's prophylaxis
crescent graft
crest
    lacrimal c., anterior
    lacrimal c., posterior
    orbital c.
cribra
    c. orbitalia of Welcker
cribral
cribrate
cribriform ligament
cribriform plate
cribriform spots
cribrum
crisis
    glaucomatocyclitic c.
    ocular c.
    oculogyric c.
    Pel's c.
crista
    c. lacrimalis anterior
    c. lacrimalis posterior
Critchett's operation
Crock encircling operation
crocodile tears
cross-action forceps
cross cylinder
cross-eye
cross-fixation
crossed amblyopia
crossed diplopia
crossed hemianopia
crossed parallax
crossed reflex
croupous conjunctivitis
crowding phenomenon
CRT screen

Additional Entries

crutch glasses
CRV (central retinal vein)
CRVO (central retinal vein occlusion)
Cryo-Barrages vitreous orbital implant
cryoextraction
cryopexy
cryophake
cryoprobe
    Rubinstein c.
cryopter
    Thomas c.
cryoretinopexy
cryotherapy
crypt
    c. of Fuchs
    c. of iris
cryptoglioma
cryptophthalmia
cryptophthalmos
cryptophthalmus
crystallin
crystalline humor
crystalline lens
crystallitis
crystalloiditis
Csapody operation
CSI daily wear
CSI T extended wear
CTL
CTL-M hydrophilic contact lens
CTL-M ocular masking contact lens (CTL)
Cuignet's method
Cuignet's test
cul-de-sac
    conjunctival c.

cup
    glaucomatous c.
    ocular c.
    ophthalmic c.
    optic c.
cup-to-disc ratio
cupped disc
cupping
    pathologic c.
cupuliform cataract
curb tenotomy
curet
    Gifford c.
    Heath c.
    Meyhoeffer c.
curvature ametropia
curvature hyperopia
curvature myopia
Cusick operation
Cusick-Sarrail operation
Custodis operation
Custodis suture
CustomEyes cosmetic contact lens (CTL)
CustomEyes hydrophilic contact lens
cutaneous horn
Cutler operation
Cutler-Beard operation
cutters
    Buettner-Parel c.
    Douvas c.
    Kloti c.
    Machemer c.
    Maguire-Harvey c.
    O'Malley-Heintz c.
    Parel-Crock c.
    Tolentino c.

Additional Entries

Cx (axis of cylindric lens)
cyanolabe
cyanosis
   c. bulbi
   c. retinae
cyclectomy
cyclic strabismus
cyclicotomy
cyclitic membrane
cyclitis
cycloanemization
cyclochoroiditis
cyclocryopexy
cyclocryotherapy
cyclodamia
cyclodialysis
cyclodiathermy
cycloduction
cycloelectrolysis
cyclogram
Cyclogyl
cyclokeratitis
Cyclomydril
cyclopentolate hydrochloride ophthalmic solution
cyclophoria
   accommodative c.
   minus c.
   negative c.

cyclophoria *(continued)*
   plus c.
   positive c.
cyclophorometer
cyclopia
cycloplegia
cycloplegic
cyclops
cycloscope
cyclospasm
cyclotropia
   minus c.
   negative c.
   plus c.
   positive c.
cycloversion
Cyl (cylindric lens or cylinder)
cylindrical lens
cyst
   pearl c.
cystic cataract
cystic eye
cystinosis
cystoid macular edema
cystotome
   von Graefe (Graefe) c.
   Wilder c.
cytomegalic inclusion disease
Czermak operation

Additional Entries

D

D (diopter)
D'ombrain operation
Dacriose
dacryadenalgia
dacryadenitis
dacryadenoscirrhus
dacryagogatresia
dacryagogic
dacryagogue
dacrycystalgia
dacrycystitis
dacryelcosis
dacryoadenalgia
dacryoadenectomy
dacryoadenitis
dacryoblennorrhea
dacryocanaliculitis
dacryocele
dacryocyst
dacryocystalgia
dacryocystectasia
dacryocystectomy
dacryocystis
dacryocystitis
dacryocystitome
dacryocystoblennorrhea
dacryocystocele
dacryocystogram
dacryocystoptosis
dacryocystorhinostenosis
dacryocystorhinostomy
dacryocystorhinotomy
dacryocystostenosis
dacryocystostomy
dacryocystosyringotomy
dacryocystotome
dacryocystotomy
dacryogenic
dacryohelcosis
dacryohemorrhea
dacryolith
dacryolithiasis
dacryoma
dacryon
dacryops
dacryopyorrhea
dacryopyosis
dacryorhinocystotomy
dacryorrhea
dacryosinusitis
dacryosolenitis
dacryostenosis
dacryosyrinx
Daily cataract needle
Daily cataract operation
Dalen-Fuchs nodules
Dalgleish operation
Dalrymple's sign
Danberg forceps
D & N (distance and near)
Daranide
dark adaptation
dark adapted
darkroom test
Daubenton's plane
Daviel operation
Daviel spoon
Davison-Geck sutures
day blindness
day sight

Additional Entries

day vision
dazzle reflex
DDH (dissociated double hypertropia)
Dean needle
Decadron
decentered
decentered spectacles
decentration
decompression of orbit
decussation
    d. of optic nerve
deep keratitis
degeneration
    Best, d. of
    disciform macular d.
    familial colloid d.
    hepatolenticular d.
    lattice d. of retina
    lenticular d.
    macular d.
    senile disciform d.
    vitelliform macular d.
    Wilson's d.
degenerative cataract
degenerative myopia
degenerative pannus
Degest 2
de Grandmont operation
Deiter's operation
DeKlair operation
de Lapersonne operation
delimiting keratotomy
dellen
Deltacon standard
deltafilcon A
deltafilcon XT lens

demecarium bromide
    ophthalmic solution
demonstration eyepiece
Demours' membrane
demyelinization
dendriform keratitis
dendritic keratitis
deorsumvergence
deorsumversion
Depo-Medrol
depression
depressor
deprimens oculi
depth
    focal d.
Derby operation
dermatochalasis
dermatoconjunctivitis
dermatomyositis
dermato-ophthalmitis
dermoid
    corneal d.
Dermostat orbital implant
Descemet's membrane
descemetitis
descemetocele
desiccation keratitis
Desmarres law
Desmarres lid clamp
Desmarres lid elevator
Desmarres lid retractor
Desmarres operation
detached vitreous
detachment
    choroidal d.
    retinal d.
deutan

Additional Entries

deuteranomalopia
deuteranomalopsia
deuteranomalous
deuteranomaly
deuteranope
deuteranopia
deuteranopic
deuteranopsia
Deutschman cataract knife
developmental cataract
deviant
    color d.
deviation
    conjugate d.
    Hering-Hellebrand d.
    heterotropic d.
    manifest d.
    minimum d.
    primary d.
    secondary d.
    skew d.
    squint d.
    strabismic d.
    tropic d.
Devic's disease
DeWecker anterior sclerotomy
DeWecker eye scissors
DeWecker iris scissors
DeWecker-Pritikin scissors
Dexacidin
Dexair
dexamethasone sodium phosphate ophthalmic solution
Dexasporin
dextroclination
dextrocular
dextrocularity
dextrocycloduction
dextroduction
dextrogyration
dextroversion
D-film
diabetic amaurosis
diabetic cataract
diabetic degenerative cataract
diabetic iritis
diabetic retinitis
diagnostic lens (Reichert)
dial
    astigmatic d.
diameter
    extracanthic d.
    intercanthic d.
diamond knife (Keeler Instruments)
Diamox
Dianoux operation
diathermy
    Mira d.
dichlorophenamide
dichromatic vision
dichromatopsia
Dickey operation
Dickey-Fox operation
Dickson Wright orbit decompression
Dicon auto perimeter 2000 (CooperVision Diagnostic Imaging)
Dieffenbach operation
diffraction
diffuse choroiditis
diffusion circle
Digilab 750 automated perimeter (Digilab)

Additional Entries

Digilab Cambridge automated perimeter (Digilab)
Digilab Model 30D (Alcon Surgical)
Digilab Model 30R (Alcon Surgical)
Digilab Model 30R/T (Alcon Surgical)
Digilab Ophthalmic
Digilab perimeter
Digilab pneumatonometer/tonographe (Digilab)
Digital B system IV
digital tonometry
diisopropyl fluorophosphate
diktyoma
Dilatair
dilate
dilation of punctum
dilator
    Hosford lacrimal d.
    Galezowski d.
Dimitry trephine
Dimmer's keratitis
diopsimeter
diopter
    prism d.
dioptometer
dioptometry
dioptoscopy
dioptre
dioptric
dioptrics
dioptrometer
dioptrometry
Dioptron V autorefractor (CooperVision Diagnostic Imaging)

dioptroscopy
dioptry
diphtheritic conjunctivitis
diplobacillary conjunctivitis
diplocoria
diplopia
    binocular d.
    crossed d.
    direct d.
    heteronymous d.
    homonymous d.
    horizontal d.
    monocular d.
    paradoxical d.
    pathological d.
    physiological d.
    torsional d.
    vertical d.
diplopiometer
diploscope
direct astigmatism
direct diplopia
direct method
direct ophthalmoscope
direct ophthalmoscopy
direct parallax
direct vision
disc
    Placido d.
disci
disciform
disciform keratitis
disciform macular degeneration
discission
    cataract, d. of
    lens, d. of
    posterior d.
discitis

Additional Entries

disclination
discoria
discus
    d. nervi optici
    d. opticus
disease
    Allbright's d.
    Basedow's d.
    Batten-Mayou d.
    Behcet's d.
    Behr's d.
    Benson's d.
    Berlin's d.
    Best's d.
    Bielchowsky-Jansky d.
    Bowen's d.
    Bright's d.
    Coats' d.
    Eales's d.
    Flajani's d.
    Flatau-Schilder d.
    flecked retina d.
    Forster's d.
    Heerfordt's d.
    Kufs' d.
    Kuhnt-Junius d.
    Leber's d.
    Norrie's d.
    Oguchi's d.
    Purtscher's d.
    Sachs' d.
    Sanders' d.
    Schilder's d.
    shipyard d.
    Spielmeyer-Vogt d.
    Stargardt's d.
    Tay-Sachs d.
    Vogt-Spielmeyer d.

disease *(continued)*
    von Hippel's d.
    von Hippel-Lindau d.
disk
    anangioid d.
    ciliary d.
    cupped d.
    gelatin d.
    micrometer d.
    optic d.
    Placido's d.
    Rekoss d.
    stenopeic d.
    stroboscopic d.
disk forceps
dislocation
    d. of the lens
disseminated choroiditis
dissociated double hypertropia
dissociated vertical deviation
distance
    angular d.
    focal d.
    infinite d.
    interocular d.
    interpupillary d.
distichia
distichiasis
distortion
distraction conus
divergence
    negative vertical d.
    positive vertical d.
divergent strabismus
divided spectacles
Docustar fundus camera (Reichert)
Doherty sphere implant

Additional Entries

doll's eye reflex
doll's eye sign
doll's head phenomenon
dominance
    ocular d.
Donaldson eyepatch
Donders' chart
Donders' glaucoma
Donders' law
Donders' line
Dorello's canal
Doryl
dot
    Mittendorf's d.
    Trantas' d.
dot hemorrhage
double homonymous hemianopsia
double hypertropia
double refraction
double vision
Douvas vitreous cutter
Doyne's familial honeycombed choroiditis
Draeger tonometer
drainage of lacrimal gland
drainage of lacrimal sac
dressing
    collodion d.
    fluffed gauze d.
    pressure d.
    Telfa d.
    Telfa plastic film d.
    tie-over d.
    wet d.
drop
    eye d.
drosopterin
Drualt's bundle
drusen
dry eye
dry-shelled cataract
D-seg
D trisomy syndrome
Duane's syndrome
Duane's test
duct
    canalicular d.
    lacrimal d.
    lacrimonasal d.
    nasal d.
    nasolacrimal d.
    tear d.
duction
ductule
    excretory d's of lacrimal gland
ductuli
    d. excretorii glandulae lacrimalis
ductulus
ductus
    d. nasolacrimalis
Duddell's membrane
Duke-Elder operation
Dunnington operation
duochrome test
Duolube
Dupuy-Dutemps dacryocystorhinostomy
Dupuy-Dutemps dacryostomy
Durasoft
Durasoft 2 (toric lens)
Durasoft 3 (toric hydrophilic lens)
Duratears

Additional Entries

Durr operation
DUSN (diffuse unilateral subacute neuroretinitis)
Duverger-Velter operation
DVD (dissociated vertical deviation)
Dvorine test
dynamic refraction
dynamic strabismus
Dynoptor ophthalmodynamometer (Reichert)
dysaptation
dyscephaly
    mandibulo-oculofacial d.
dyschromasia
dyschromatopsia
dyscoria
dyskeratosis
    hereditary benign intraepithelial d.
dyskeratotic
dyslexia
dysmegalopsia
dysmetria
dysmetropsia
dysmorphopsia
dysopia
    d. algera
dysopsia
dysplasia
    encephalo-ophthalmic d.
    oculoauricular d.
    oculoauriculovertebral d.
    oculodentodigital d.
    ophthalmomandibulomelic d.
dysplastic
dystonia
    d. lenticularis
dystrophia
    d. adiposa corneae
    d. endothelialis
    d. epithelialis corneae
dystrophy
    corneal d.
    Fuchs' d.
    granular corneal (Groenouw's type I) d.
    lattice d.
    macular corneal d.
    papoculocerebrorenal d.
    progressive tapetochoroidal d.
    Salzmann's nodular corneal d.
    tapetochoroidal d.

Additional Entries

Additional Entries

E

Eales's disease
E carpine
ECCE (extracapsular cataract extraction)
eccentric limitation
echinophthalmia
echography
echo-ophthalmography
echothiophate iodide
eclipse scotoma
Econochlor
Econopred
Econopred Plus
ectasia
    corneal e.
    scleral e.
ectoderm
ectodermatosis
ectodermosis
ectopia
    e. iridis
    e. lentis
    e. pupillae congenita
ectopic
ectropion
    cicatricial e.
    flaccid e.
    paralytic e.
    pigment layer, e. of
    sarcomatosum, e.
    senilis, e.
    spasticum, e.
    uvea, e.
ectropionize
ectropium

eczematous conjunctivitis
edema
    Berlin's e.
    periretinal e.
edetate disodium
Edinger-Westphal nucleus
edrophonium chloride
Edward's syndrome
effect
    Braid e.
efferent nerve
efficiency
    visual e.
egilops
Egyptian conjunctivitis
Ehlers-Danlos syndrome
Ehrmann's test
eidetic
eidoptometry
EKC (epidemic keratoconjunctivitis)
Eldridge-Green lamp
electric cataract
electrodiagnosis
electrodiaphake
electromagnetic spectrum
electronystagmograph
electronystagmography
electro-oculogram (EOG)
electro-oculography
electroparacentesis
electroperimetry
electroretinogram (ERG)
electroretinograph
electroretinography

Additional Entries

elephantiasis
    e. oculi
elevation
ELISA (enzyme-linked immunosorbent assay)
Elliott corneal trephine
Elschnig blepharorrhaphy
Elschnig bodies
Elschnig canthorrhaphy
Elschnig cataract knife
Elschnig forceps
Elschnig iridectomy
Elschnig keratoplasty
Elschnig pearls
Elschnig spatula
embolism
    retinal e.
embryonal nuclear cataract
embryotoxon
    anterior e.
    posterior e.
emergent ray
emergency light reflex
eminence
    postchiasmatic e.
emmetropia
emmetropic
emmetropic eye
encephalofacial angiomatosis
encephalo-ophthalmic dysplasia
encephalopathy
    Wernicke's e.
encirclement of the globe
encircling for scleral buckle
endocrine exophthalmos
endogenous uveitis
endophthalmitis
    e. phaco-allergica

endophthalmite *(continued)*
    e. phaco-anaphylactica
    e. phacogenetica
endothelium
    camerae anterioris bulbi, e.
    camerae anterioris oculi, e.
    corneal e.
endpoint nystagmus
enophthalmos
Enroth's sign
enstrophe
entiris
entochoroidea
entocornea
entophthalmia
entoptic
entoptoscope
entoptoscopy
entoretina
entropion
    cicatrical e.
    Hotz e.
    spastic e.
entropionize
entropium
enucleate
enucleated
enucleation
Enuclene
enzyme glaucoma
EOG (electro-oculogram)
EOM (extraocular muscle)
eopsia
epiblepharon
epibulbar
epicanthal
epicanthal skin fold
epicanthic

Additional Entries

epicanthine
epicanthine fold
epicanthus
   e. inversus
epicapsular lens star
epicorneascleritis
epidemic blindness
epidemic conjunctivitis
epidemic keratoconjunctivitis (EKC)
Epifrin
E-Pilo-1
E-Pilo-2
E-Pilo-3
E-Pilo-4
E-Pilo-6
Epinal
epinephrine bitartrate ophthalmic solution
epiphora
episclera
episcleral
episcleral arteries
episcleral lamina
episcleritis
episclerotitis
epitarsus
epithelial
epitheliosis
   e. desquamativa conjunctivae
epithelium
   anterior e. of cornea
   corneal e.
   lens, e. of
epizootic keratoconjunctivitis
Eppy/N
Epstein collar stud acrylic lens implant

equator
   e. of eyeball
   e. of lens
equatorial
equatorial staphyloma
equilateral hemianopia
equilibrating operation
Erbakan operation
ERG (electroretinogram)
erroneous projection
erysiphake
   Bell e.
   Harrington e.
   Maumenee-Park e.
erythema multiforme
erythrochloropia
erythrochloropsia
erythrolabe
erythromycin
erythropsia
Escapini operation
escorcin
eserine
esophoria (E)
esophoric
esotropia (ET)
   clock mechanism e.
esotropic
essential blepharospasm
Esser operation
Esser eyelid operation
esthesiophysiology
esthesodic
ET (esotropia)
etafilcon A
Ethamide
Ethilon sutures
ethmoid canal

Additional Entries

ethoxzolamide
E trisomy
eucatropine hydrochloride
euchromatopsy
euphoropsia
euryopia
euryphotic
euthyscope
evagination
    optic e.
Everbusch ptosis operation
evisceration
evisceration of eyeball
evulsio
    e. nervi optici
evulsion
E-W (Edinger-Westphal)
  nucleus
Ewing operation
excavatio
    e. disci
    e. papillae nervi optici
excavation
    atrophic e.
    glaucomatous e.
    physiologic e.
excessive accommodation
excision of lacrimal gland
excision of lacrimal sac
exciting eye
excycloduction
excyclophoria
excyclotropia
excyclovergence
Executive bifocal lens
exenteration of orbital contents
exfoliation
exocataphoria

exodeviation
exophoria (X)
exophoric
exophthalmic
exophthalmic goiter
exophthalmic ophthalmoplegia
exophthalmogenic
exophthalmometer
exophthalmometric
exophthalmometry
exophthalmos
    endocrine e.
    malignant e.
    ophthalmoplegic e.
    pulsating e.
    thyrotoxic e.
    thyrotropic e.
exophthalmos-producing
  substance
exorbitism
exotropia (XT) *V-pattern*
    basic e.
    consecutive e.
    convergence insufficiency e.
    divergence excess e.
    intermittent e.
    secondary e.
    sensory e.
exotropic
exposure keratitis
expulsive hemorrhage
extended wear lens
Extenzyme
external axis of eye
external hordeolum
external ophthalmopathy
external pterygoid-levator
  synkinesis

Additional Entries

external strabismus
extorsion
extracanthic diameter
extracapsular extraction of cataract
extraciliary fibers
extraction
    e. of a cataract
extractor
    Krwawicz cataract e.
extraocular muscles
extraoculogram
extravisual zone
extrinsic muscles
extrusion needle
exudative choroiditis
exudative retinitis
exudative retinopathy
eye
    blear e.
    Bright's e.
    cinema e.
    compound e.
    crossed e.
    cystic e.
    dark-adapted e.
    exciting e.
    fixating e.
    Fox e.
    hare's e.
    hop e.
    Klieg e.
    light-adapted e.
    monochromatic e.
    Nairobi e.
    pink e.
    primary e.
    reduced e.

eye *(continued)*
    schematic e.
    secondary e.
    shipyard e.
    Snellen's reform e.
    sympathizing e.
    wall e.
eyeball compression reflex
eyeball-heart reflex
eyebank specular microscope
eyebrow
eyecup
eye-ear plane
eyeglass
eyeground
eyelash
eyelid
eyelid closure reflex
eyelid anatomy
    aponeurosis
    canthus
    caruncula
    ciliary margins
    conjunctiva
    fibers of orbicularis oculi
    fornix
    inferior tarsus
    lacrimal ducts
    lacrimal sac
    lacus lacrimalis
    lamina
    lateral canthus
    levator palpebrae superioris
    medial palpebral ligament
    meibomian glands
    Muller muscle
    nasojugal
    nasolacrimal duct

Additional Entries

eyelid anatomy *(continued)*
    orbital margins
    orbital septum
    palpebral fissure
    palpebral furrow
    palpebral raphe
    palpebrarum
    plica semilunaris
    posterior lamina
    Riolan's muscle
    superior fornix
    superior tarsus
    tarsal glands
    tarsal muscles
    tarsal plate
    tarsus
    tarsus orbital septum
    tunica conjunctiva
Eye-Pak drape

eyepiece
    comparison e.
    compensating e.
    demonstration e.
    huygenian e.
    negative e.
    positive e.
    Ramsden's e.
    widefield e.
eyepoint
eye shield
eye speculum
eye spot
eyestrain
Eye-Stream
eyeturn
eye wash
Eye-Zine

Additional Entries

F

Fabry's disease
facial (VII) nerve
facial vision
facies
    f. anterior lentis
    f. anterior palpebrarum
    f., Hutchinson's
    f. orbitalis alae magnae
    f. orbitalis alae majoris
    f. orbitalis ossis frontalis
    f. orbitalis ossis zygomatici
    f. posterior corneae
    f. posterior iridis
    f. posterior lentis
    f. posterior palpebrarum
factor
    diffusion f.
    spreading f.
facultative hyperopia
facultative suppression
faculty
    fusion f.
Faden procedure
falciform fold
false image
false macula
false ptosis
false vision
familial colloid degeneration
Fanta operation
fantascope
Farber's lipogranulomatosis
farinata
Farnsworth D15 test
Farnsworth D100 test
far point
far point of convergence
far sight
Fasanella-Servat operation
fascia
    ff. musculares bulbi
    ff. musculares oculi
    ff. of eye, muscular
    ff., orbital
    ff. orbitales
fascia lata sling
fascia musculares bulbi
fasciae musculares oculi
fasciae orbitales
fascicular keratitis
fascicular ophthalmoplegia
fatty exudate
fc (footcandles)
Federoff four loop iris clip lens implant
Federoff Type I lens implant
Federoff Type II lens implant
Fergus operation
Ferree-Rand perimeter
Ferrein's canal
FFF fields
fiber
    accessory f.
    Berneheimer's f.
    circular f's of ciliary muscle
    chief f.
    cilioequatorial f.
    cilioposterocapsular f.
    cone f.

Additional Entries

fiber *(continued)*
    continuous f.
    corticonuclear f.
    extraciliary f.
    Gratiolet's radiating f.
    interciliary f.
    main f.
    meridional f's of ciliary muscle
    Muller's f.
    orbiculoanterocapsular f.
    orbiculociliary f.
    orbiculoposterocapsular f.
    Ritter's f.
    Sappey's f.
    von Monakow's f.
    zonular f.
fiberoptic pic
fibers of lens
fibers of orbicularis oculi
fibra
fibrae
    f. circulares musculi ciliaris
    f. lentis
    f. meridionales
    f. meridionales musculi ciliaris
    f. zonulares
fibroid cataract
fibroplasia
    retrolental f.
fibrous dysplasia
fibrous tunic of eyeball
Fick's axes
Fick's halo
field
    cribriform f. of vision
    fixation, f. of

field *(continued)*
    Forel's f.
    H2 f.
    overshot f. of vision
    surplus f.
    visual f.
figure
    Stifel's f.
filamentary keratitis
Filatov keratoplasty
Filatov-Marzinkowsky operation
filter
    Wrattan #47 f.
filtering bleb
filtering cicatrix
filtering operation
filtration angle
fine dissecting forceps
finger vision
Fink cataract operation
Fink hook
fish mouth tear
Fisher-Arlt forceps
Fisons Corporation
fissura
    f. orbitalis inferior
    f. orbitalis superior
fissure
    choroid f.
    corneal f.
    orbital f., inferior
    orbital f., superior
    sphenoidal f.
    sphenoidal f., inferior
    sphenoidal f., superior
    sphenomaxillary f.
    sphenoccipital f.

Additional Entries

fistula
    cornea, f.
    lacrimal f.
fixate
fixating eye
fixation
    binocular f.
fixation point
fixed pupil
flaccid ectropion
Flajani's disease
Flajani's operation
flare
flash keratoconjunctivitis
flashes of light
flat cornea
Flatau-Schilder disease
flattest meridian
flecked retina disease
Fleischer ring
Flexlens
Flexlens custom soft lens (Flexlens)
Flexsol
Flieringa ring
flight blindness
floaters
Florentine iris
floriform cataract
floriform developmental cataract
Floropryl
Flow System Model 613 (Surgical Design)
fluffed gauze dressing
fluid cataract
Fluoracaine
fluorescein angiography
fluorescence retinal photography
Fluorescite
Fluoresoft
Fluor-I-Strip
Fluor-I-Strip A.T.
fluorophotometry
Fluoropryl
Fluress
FML
FML Forte
focal depth
focal distance
focal interval
focal point
foci
    principal f.
focus
    aplanatic f.
    conjugate f.
    real f.
    virtual f.
Foerster-Fuchs' spot
fogging
fold
    ciliary f.
    conjunctival f.
    epicanthal f.
    epicanthine f.
    Hasner's f.
    palpebral f.
    retrotarsal f.
follicle
follicular conjunctivitis
follicular iritis
Foltz's valve
Fontana's spaces
foot-candle

Additional Entries

foot-lambert
foramen
    Bozzi's f.
    inferior zygomatic f.
    infraorbital f.
    infraorbitale, f.
    lacerate f., anterior
    lacerate f., middle
    lacerum anterius, f.
    optic f. of sphenoid bone
    optic f. of sclera
    opticus ossis, f.
    orbitomalar f.
    Soemmering's f.
    sphenoidalis f.
    supraorbital f.
    supraorbitale, f.
    supraorbitalis, f.
    zygomatic f.
    zygomatic f., inferior
    zygomatic f. of Arnold, internal
    zygomatic f., orbital
    zygomatic f., posterior
    zygomatic f., superior
    zygomaticoorbital f.
    zygomaticoorbitale, f.
foramina
forced duction test
forceps
    Arruga capsule f.
    Ayer f.
    Baird f.
    Barraquer f.
    Bonn f.
    Botvin f.
    Bracken f.
    Castroviejo f.
    Castroviejo suture f.
    Castroviejo-Arruga f.
    Chandler f.
    Citelli f.
    Colibri f.
    Danberg f.
    disk f.
    dissecting f.
    Elschnig f.
    fine f.
    Fisher-Arlt f.
    Forster f.
    Francis f.
    Gifford f.
    Gill-Hess iris f.
    Girard f.
    Halsted curved mosquito f.
    Hubbard f.
    Hunt f.
    Katzin-Barraquer f.
    Kelman f.
    Kerrison f.
    Kirby f.
    Knapp f.
    Lambert f.
    Lister f.
    Lordan f.
    Max Fine f.
    McCullough f.
    McCullough suture-tying f.
    McGuire f.
    McLean f.
    Moehle f.
    O'Brien f.
    Prince f.
    Quevedo f.
    Reese f.
    roller f.

Additional Entries

forceps *(continued)*
    Schweigger f.
    Smart f.
    Takahashi f.
    Thorpe f.
    Verhoeff f.
    von Graefe iris f.
    Worth f.
forehead
    bony f.
Forel's field
fornix
    f. conjunctivae inferior
    f. conjunctivae superior
    f. sacci
    f. lacrimalis
Forssman's carotid syndrome
Forster's choroiditis
Forster's disease
Forster's forceps
Forster's photometer
Forster's snare
fossa
    hyaloid f.
    lacrimal f.
    lenticular f.
fossae
Foster-Kennedy syndrome
Fould operation
fovea
    central f. of retina
    trochlear f.
foveal vision
foveola
Foville's syndrome
Fox aluminum eye shield
Fox conformer
Fox operation
Fox eye shield
Fox eyelid implant
fpa (far point of accommodation)
fracture
    blow-out f.
Fragmatome Model 8300 (CooperVision Surgical)
Fragmatome system
frame
    trial f.
framework
    scleral f.
    uveal f.
framing
Franceschetti corepraxy
Franceschetti keratoplasty
Francis forceps
Francois syndrome
Frankfort horizontal plane
Fraunhofer's lines
free margin of eyelid
Frelex
Fresnel lens
Frey tunneled implant
Fricke eyelid operation
Friede operation
Friedenwald-Guyton operation
Friedman clip
Frigitronics
Frigitronics binocular indirect ophthalmoscope, incandescent (Frigitronics)
Frigitronics nitrous oxide cryosurgery apparatus
frons
    f. of cranium
frontal

Additional Entries

frontal triangle
frontal tuber
frontolacrimal suture
Frost suture
Frost-Lang operation
Fuchs dystrophy
Fuchs operation
Fuchs coloboma
Fukala operation
Ful-Glo
Ful-Vue ophthalmoscope (Reichert)
Ful-Vue spot retinoscope (Reichert)
Ful-Vue streak retinoscope (Reichert)
functional blindness
fundus
    albinotic f.
    tessellated f.
    tigroid f.
fundus albipunctatus
fundus camera FF 4 (Carl Zeiss)
fundus camera FK 30 (Carl Zeiss)
fundus flavimaculatus
fundus microscopy
fundus/retinal camera
Funduscein
funduscope
funduscopy
funnel
    muscular f.
    vascular f.
furrow
    scleral f.
furrow keratitis
Fusarium
fusiform cataract
fusion
    binocular f.
fusion faculty
fusion tubes
fusional convergence
Fyoderov lens

Additional Entries

G

Gaillard operation
Gaillard-Arlt suture
galactosemia
galeropia
galeropsia
Galezowski lacrimal dilator
gamma angle
ganglion
    ciliary g.
    ophthalmic g.
    optic orbital g.
    Schacher's g.
ganglion cell layer
ganglionic layer of optic nerve
ganglionic layer of retina
ganglionic stratum of optic nerve
ganglionic stratum of retina
ganglionitis
    acute posterior g.
gangliosidoses
Gantrisin
Garamycin
Garcia-Novito eye implant
gargoylism
gas
    tear g.
gas permeable lens starter system (Barnes-Hind)
Gass cannula
Gaucher's disease
Gaul's pits
Gayet operation
gaze
gaze nystagmus

gelatin disk
Gel Clean
Gelfilm retinal orbital implant
Gel Flex lens
general cataract
generalized xanthelasma
Genesis 4 contact lens, soft
Geneva lens clock
geniculate body
geniculo-calcarine tract
Genoptic
Gentacidin
Gentafair
Gentak
gentamicin
Georgariou operation
gerontotoxon
gerontoxon
ghost ophthalmoscope
giant papillary conjunctivitis (GPC)
Giemsa stain
Gierke's disease
Gifford curet
Gifford forceps
Gifford keratotomy
Gifford operation
Gifford sign
Gill blade
Gill knife
Gill needle
Gill scissors
Gill-Hess forceps
Gillies operation
Gills-Welsh style handpiece

Additional Entries

Girard forceps
Girard keratoprosthesis
Giraud-Teulon law
glabella
glabellad
glabellum
gland
    Baumgarten's g.
    Bruch's g.
    Ciaccio's g.
    ciliary g.
    ciliary g. of conjunctiva
    conjunctival g.
    Harder's g.
    harderian g.
    Henle's g.
    Krause's g.
    lacrimal g.
    lacrimal g's, accessory
    Manz' g.
    Moll's g's
    Rosenmuller's g.
    sebaceous g's of conjunctiva
    trachoma g.
    Waldeyer's g.
    Wolfring, g. of
    Zeis, g. of
glandula
    g. lacrimalis inferior
    g. lacrimalis superior
glandulae
    g. ciliares
    g. ciliares conjunctivales
    g. conjunctivales
    g. lacrimales accessoriae
    g. mucosae conjunctivae
    g. sebaceae
glare

glarometer
glass
    watch g.
glassblower's cataract
glasses
    bifocal g.
    contact g.
    crutch g.
    Hallauer's g.
    hyperbolic g.
    snow g.
    sun g.
    trifocal g.
glass lens
glaucoma
    absolute g.
    acute congestive g.
    air-block g.
    angle-closure g.
    angle-recession g.
    aphakic g.
    apoplectic g.
    auricular g.
    capsular g.
    chronic narrow-angle g.
    chronic simple g.
    ciliary block g.
    closed-angle g.
    congenital g.
    congestive g.
    Donders' g.
    enzyme g.
    hemorrhagic g.
    infantile g.
    inflammatory g.
    juvenile g.
    lenticular g.
    malignant g.

Additional Entries

glaucoma *(continued)*
  narrow-angle g.
  neovascular g.
  noncongestive g.
  obstructive g.
  open-angle g.
  phakogenic g.
  phakolytic g.
  pigmentary g.
  primary g.
  secondary g.
  simple g.
  traumatic g.
  vitreous-block g.
  wide-angle g.
glaucomatocyclitic crisis
glaucomatous
glaucomatous cataract
glaucomatous cup
glaucomatous excavation
glaucomatous habit
glaucomatous halo
glaucomatous ring
Glaucon
glaucosis
glioma
  g. endophytum
  g. exophytum
  g. optic
  g. retinae
gliomatosis
gliomatous
gliosarcoma
  g. retinae
globe
globule
  Morgagni's g.
globuli

glycerin
gnat
  eye g.
goblet cells
goiter
  exophthalmic g.
Goldenhar's syndrome
Goldman serrated knife
Goldmann applanation tonometer
Goldmann-Larsson operation
Goldmann multi-mirrored lens implant
Goldmann perimeter
Goldmann three mirror lens implant
Goldstein lacrimal sac retractor
Golgi type I neurons
Golgi type II neurons
Gomez-Marquez operation
Gonak
Gonin cautery
goniolens
goniophotocoagulation
goniopuncture
gonioscope
gonioscopic prism solution
gonioscopy
Goniosol
goniosynechia
goniotomy
gonoblennorrhea
gonococcal conjunctivitis
gonorrheal conjunctivitis
gouty iritis
GP-II contact lenses (Barnes-Hind)
GPC (giant papillary conjunctivitis)

Additional Entries

Gradenigo's syndrome
Gradle keratoplasty
Gradle trephine
Graefe cataract knife (von Graefe)
Graefe's disease
Graefe's knife
Graefe's operation
Graefe's sign
Graefe's test
graft
    corneal g.
    lamellar g.
granular conjunctivitis
granular corneal dystrophy (Groenouw's type I)
granule
    cone g.
    rod g.
granulomatous uveitis
graphoscope
Gratiolet's radiating fibers
grattage
Graves' disease
gravidic retinitis
gray cataract
GRC-WT fundus camera
greater ring of iris
Greaves operation
green blindness
green cataract
Green cataract knife
Green double spatula
Green iris replacer
greyish-white corneal scar
Gridley intraocular lens
Grieshaber trephine
Grimsdale operation
Groenouw's dystrophy
Gronblad-Strandberg syndrome
groove
    Blessig's g.
    lacrimal g.
    nasolacrimal g.
    optic g.
    Verga's g.
gross tereopsis
Grossmann's operation
Gruning's magnet
gtt. (drop or drops)
guanethidine
Guibor's chart
guillotine cutting tip
Guist scissors
Guist sphere implant
Gullstrand's law
Gullstrand's slit lamp
Gunn dots
Gunn pupil
Gunn syndrome
gutta
    g. serena
guttata
Gutzeit operation
Guyton operation
Guyton-Park lid speculum
gyrate atrophy

Additional Entries

H

H (hyperphoria)
Haab's magnet
Haab's reflex
Haag-Streit slit lamp
habit
    glaucomatous h.
Haenel symptom
Hague cataract lamp
Halberg clip
Haidinger's brush
Haik eye implant
halation
Halberstraedter-Prowazek bodies
half vision
half-retinal
Hallauer's glasses
Hallermann-Streiff syndrome
Hallermann-Streiff-Francois syndrome
Haller's layer
halo
    Fick's h.
    glaucomatous h.
    senile h.
halo symptom
halo vision
Halpin's operation
Halsted curved mosquito forceps
hamartoma
hamular process of lacrimal bone
hand movement test
Hand-Schuller-Christian disease
Hannover's canal

haploscope
    mirror h.
haploscopic
haploscopic vision
haptic area lens implant
Harada Ito procedure
Harada's syndrome
hard cataract
Harder's glands
harderian glands
Hardy-Rand-Ritter test charts
hare's eye
Harman operation
harmonious retinal correspondence
Harms-Dannheim operation
Harrington erysiphake
Harrington-Flocks test
Harrison retractor
Hasner's fold
Hasner's lid
Hasner's valve
Hassall-Henle bodies
HCL (hard contact lens)
Healon
heat degenerative cataract
Heath curet
heat-ray cataract
hedger's cataract
Heerfordt's disease
Heidenhaim's syndrome
Heijl-Krakau screening
Heine cyclodialysis
Heisrath's operation
helpharoadenitis

Additional Entries

___
___
___
___
___

hemangioma
hemeralopia
hemiachromatopsia
hemiamaurosis
hemiamblyopia
hemianopia
    absolute h.
    altitudinal h.
    bilateral h.
    binasal h.
    binocular h.
    bitemporal h.
    complete h.
    congruous h.
    crossed h.
    equilateral h.
    heteronymous h.
    homonymous h.
    horizontal h.
    incomplete h.
    incongruous h.
    lateral h.
    lower h.
    nasal h.
    quadrant h.
    quadrantic h.
    relative h.
    temporal h.
    true h.
    unilateral h.
    uniocular h.
    upper h.
    vertical h.
hemianopic
hemianopsia
    altitudinal h.
hemianoptic
hemianoptic scotoma
hemichromatopsia
hemiopalgia
hemiopia
hemiopic
hemiopic pupillary reaction
hemiscotosis
hemisphere perimeters
hemophthalmia
hemophthalmos
hemophthalmus
hemorrhage
    dot h.
    expulsive h.
hemorrhagic glaucoma
Henle's fiber layer
Henle's glands
hepatolenticular degeneration
heptachromic
Herbert's pits
hereditary benign intraepithelial
    dyskeratosis syndrome
hereditary progressive
    arthro-ophthalmopathy
Hering-Hellebrand deviation
Hering's law
Hering's test
Hering's theory
herpes
    h. corneae
    h. ocular
    h. zoster ophthalmicus
herpes keratitis
herpetic keratitis
Herplex
Hess eyelid operation
Hess-Lees screen
Hess ptosis operation
Hess screen test

Additional Entries

Hess spoon
heterochromia
    h. iridis
heterochromic cataract
heterochromic iridocyclitis
heterochromic uveitis
heteronymous diplopia
heteronymous hemianopia
heteronymous image
heteronymous parallax
heterophoria
heterophoric
heterophthalmia
heterophthalmos
heteropsia
heteroptics
heteroscopy
heterotrophy
heterotropia
    comitant h.
    concomitant h.
    paralytic h.
hexachromic
Hiff operation
high contrast
Hildreth cautery and tip
Hippel's disease
hippus
Hirschberg's magnet
Hirschberg's method
Hirschberg's test
Hirschman spatula
histo spots
HM (hand movements)
HM/3 ft (hand motion at 3 ft)
Hogan dacryostomy
Hogan keratoplasty
Hollenhorst plaques

hollow sphere orbital implant
Holmgren test
Holth iridencleisis
Holth punch sclerectomy
homatropine hydrobromide
    ophthalmic solution
Homen's syndrome
homocystinuria
homonymous
homonymous diplopia
homonymous hemianopia
homonymous hemianopsia
homonymous image
homonymous parallax
Honan cuff
hook
    Fink h.
    Jaeger h.
    Jameson muscle h.
    McReynolds h.
    Scobee h.
    Sinskey h.
    Tyrrell h.
    von Graefe h.
Horay operation
hordeolum
horizontal diplopia
horizontal hemianopia
horizontal strabismus
Horner's law
Horner's muscle
Horner's ptosis
Horner's pupil
Horner's syndrome
Horner-Bernard syndrome
horopter
    Vieth-Muller h.
horopteric

Additional Entries

horseshoe tear
Horvath operation
Hosford lacrimal dilator
Hoskins & Birks instruments
Hotz entropion operation
Hovius' canal
Hovius' circle
Hovius' membrane
Hovius' plexus
HRR test
Hruby contact lens implant
HSV (herpes simplex virus)
HT (hypertropia)
Hubbard forceps
Hudson-Stahli line
hue
Hueck's ligament
Hughes eye implant
Hughes eyelid operation
Hummelsheim procedure
humor
    aqueous h.
    crystalline h.
    ocular h.
    plasmoid h.
    vitreous h.
Humorsol
Humphrey autokeratometer
Humphrey automatic refractor (HAR)
Humphrey field analyzer (Allergan Humphrey)
Humphrey lens analyzer Model 306 (Allergan Humphrey)
Humphrey ultrasonic biometer
Humphrey ultrasonic pachometer
Hunt forceps

Hunter's syndrome
Hunter-Hurler syndrome
Hunt-Transley operation
Hurler's syndrome
Huschke's valve
Hutchinson's disease
Hutchinson's facies
Hutchinson's pupil
huygenian
huygenian eyepiece
hyaline
hyalinization
hyalitis
    asteroid h.
    punctate h.
    suppurative h.
hyalogen
hyaloid
hyaloid fossa
hyaloideocapsular ligament
hyaloiditis
hyalonyxis
hyaluronic acid
hyaluronidase
Hyazyme
hydatoid
Hydeltrasol
Hydracon (contact lens, soft)
Hydracon toric (contact lens, soft)
hydroblepharon
hydrocortisone acetate ophthalmic suspension
Hydrocurve extended wear soft lenses
Hydrocurve II bifocal contact lenses (Barnes-Hind)
hydrodiascope

Additional Entries

hydrodictiotomy
Hydromarc
Hydron Custom toric contact lens, soft
Hydron hydrophilic contact lenses (American Hydron)
Hydron Mini contact lens, soft
Hydron spincast contact lens, soft
Hydron X-70 contact lens, soft
Hydron Z plus contact lens, soft
Hydron Zero T contact lens, soft
Hydron Zero 4 contact lens, soft
Hydron Zero 4F contact lens, soft
Hydron Zero 6 contact lens, soft
Hydronol
hydrophthalmos
    h. anterior
    h. posterior
    h. totalis
hydrophthalmus
hydrops
HydroSight (contact lens, soft)
HydroSight Thin (contact lens, soft)
hydroxyamphetamine hydrobromide ophthalmic solution
hygroblepharic
hyperbolic glasses
hyperemia
hyperesthesia
    optic h.
hypereuryopia
hyperfluorescence
hyperlipoproteinemia
hypermature cataract
hypermetropia
hypermetropic astigmatism
hyperophthalmopathic syndrome
hyperopia
    absolute h.
    axial h.
    curvature h.
    facultative h.
    index h.
    latent h.
    manifest h.
    refractive h.
    relative h.
    total h.
hyperopic astigmatism
hyperoxophoria
hyperphoria
hypertelorism
    ocular h.
    orbital h.
hypertensive neuroretinopathy
hypertensive retinitis
hypertonic saline
hypertropia (HT)
hyphema
hypocyclosis
hypofluorescence
hypophoria
hypophysis
hypoplastic
hypopyon
hypopyon keratitis
hyposcleral
Hypotears
hypotelorism
    ocular h.
    orbital h.

Additional Entries

hypotonia
   h. oculi
hypotropia

hypsiconchous
hysteric amaurosis
hysteric amblyopia

Additional Entries

I

I/A handpiece (Contemporary Surgical)
I/A Vitrophage-Peyman Unit (Cilco)
ianthinopsia
ICCE (intracapsular cataract extraction)
ICD (intercanthal distance)
idioretinal
idioretinal light
idoxuridine ophthalmic solution
IDU (idoxuridine)
IIB slit lamp (Marco)
III slit lamp (Marco)
IK (interstitial keratitis)
I-Knife (Alcon Surgical)
Iliff exenteration
Iliff ptosis operation
Iliff-Haus operation
illacrimation
illaqueation
illusion
    Kuhnt's i.
    passive i.
image
    accidental i.
    false i.
    heteronymous i.
    homonymous i.
    incidental i.
    mirror i.
    negative i.
    ocular i.
    optical i.
    Purkinje i.

image *(continued)*
    Purkinje-Sanson i.
    retinal i.
    Sanson's i.
    specular i.
    visual i.
immature cataract
implant
    acrylic i.
    Allen i.
    Allen-Braley i.
    Arruga i.
    Arruga-Moura-Brazil i.
    aspheric i.
    Barkan infant i.
    Barraquer i.
    Berens i.
    Berens-Rosa scleral i.
    Binkhorst collar stud i.
    Boberg-Ans i.
    Bonaccolto monoplex i.
    Brawner i.
    Brown-Dohlman corneal i.
    Cardona focalizing fundus i.
    Cardona gonio-focalizing i.
    Castroviejo acrylic i.
    Choyce i.
    Cogan-Boberg-Ans i.
    Cryo-Barrages vitreous i.
    Dermostat i.
    Doherty sphere i.
    Donnheim i.
    Epstein collar stud acrylic i.
    Federoff four loop iris clip i.
    Federoff Type I i.

Additional Entries
_____
_____
_____
_____
_____

implant *(continued)*
- Federoff Type II i.
- Fox sphere i.
- Frey tunneled i.
- Garcia-Novito eye i.
- Gelfilm retinal i.
- Goldmann multi-mirrored i.
- Goldmann three mirror i.
- Guist sphere i.
- Haik eye i.
- haptic area i.
- hollow sphere i.
- Hruby contact i.
- Hughes eye i.
- Iowa i.
- Jordan i.
- King i.
- Koeppe gonioscopic i.
- Kryptok bifocals i.
- Landegger i.
- Lemoine eye i.
- Levitt eye i.
- Lincoff i.
- Lovac six mirror gonioscopic i.
- lucite sphere i.
- Lyda Ivalon-Lucite i.
- Melauskas i.
- Mulberger i.
- Mules sphere i.
- Nocito eye i.
- O'Malley self-adhering i.
- Plexiglas i.
- polyethylene sphere i.
- Radin-Rosenthal eye i.
- Ridley anterior chamber i.
- Ridley Mark II i.
- Rodin i.

implant *(continued)*
- Rosa-Berens i.
- Ruedemann eye i.
- Ruiz Plano fundus i.
- Schepens hollow hemisphere i.
- shell i.
- Sichi i.
- Silastic i.
- silicone meshed motility i.
- Smith orbital floor i.
- solid silicone with Supramid mesh i.
- Strampelli i.
- Teflon orbital floor i.
- Troncosco tubular gonioscopic i.
- Troutman magnetic i.
- Ultex i.
- Uribe i.
- VA magnetic i.
- Varigray i.
- Varilux i.
- Volk conoid i.
- Walter Reed i.

impression tonometer
Imre keratoplasty
Imre canthoplasty
Imre flap operation
Imre lid operation
incidental color
incidental image
incipient cataract
incisura
- i. ethmoidalis ossis frontalis
- i. frontalis
- i. lacrimalis

Additional Entries

incisura *(continued)*
    i. maxillae
    i. supraorbitalis
incisurae
incisure
    ethmoidal i.
    ethmoidal i. of frontal bone
    frontal i.
    lacrimal i. of maxilla
    supraorbital i.
inclusion conjunctivitis
incomitant strabismus
incomplete hemianopia
incongruous
incongruous hemianopia
incontinentia pigmenti
incycloduction
incyclophoria
incyclotropia
inclyclovergence
indentation for retinal tear
indentation tonometer
index
    cephalo-orbital i.
    orbital i. of Broca
index ametropia
index hyperopia
index myopia
indirect ophthalmoscope
indirect ophthalmoscopy
indirect vision
infantile cataract
infantile glaucoma
infectious ophthalmoplegia
inferior canaliculus
inferior fasiculus
inferior orbital fissure
inferior tarsus
infinite distance
Inflamase
Inflamase Forte
inflammatory glaucoma
infraduction
infranuclear pathway
infraorbital
infraorbital arteries
infraorbital canal
infraorbital foramen
infraorbital margin of maxilla
infraorbital margin of orbit
infraorbital nerve
infrapalpebral sulcus
infraversion
injection
    circumcorneal i.
    Van Lint type i.
inlet
input nerve
InnoMed Corporation
InnoMed glaretester
InnoMed Terry keratometer
INNOVA laser tube
insufficiency
    i. of the eyelids
intercalary staphyloma
intercanthic diameter
interciliary fibers
interlamellar spaces
Intermedics intraocular lens
Intermedics intraocular radius gauge
Intermedics phaco and I/A kits (Intermedics Intraocular)
intermittent exotropia
intermittent strabismus
intermittent tropia

Additional Entries

internal axis of eye
internal ophthalmopathy
internal strabismus
internuclear ophthalmoplegia
internuclear paralysis
interocular distance
interorbital
interpalpebral
interpalpebral zone
interpupillary
interpupillary distance
Inter-Sharp micro scalpel (Intermedics Intraocular)
Intersol
interstitial keratitis
intervaginal spaces of optic nerve
interval
    focal i.
    Sturm's i.
intorsion
intoxication amaurosis
intracapsular
intracapsular extraction of cataract
intraepithelial epithelioma
intraocular
intraocular pressure (IOP)
intraocular tension
intraorbital
intraretinal
intrascleral
intrasheath tenotomy
intrinsic light
introducer
    Carter sphere i.
intumescent cataract
inverse astigmatism

IO (inferior oblique)
IOCARE balanced salt
IOCARE I/A procedure pack
IOCARE titanium needles (Iolab)
iodopsin
IOL (intraocular lens)
IOLAB Corporation
IOLAB intraocular lens
ION (ischemic optic neuropathy)
IOP (intraocular pressure)
IOPTEX intraocular lens
Iowa orbital implant
IPD (interpupillary distance)
ipsilateral
IR (inferior rectus)
iridal
iridalgia
iridauxesis
iridectasis
iridectome
iridectomesodialysis
iridectomize
iridectomy
    optic i.
    optical i.
    peripheral i.
    preliminary i.
    preparatory i.
    stenopeic i.
    therapeutic i.
iridectopia
iridectropium
iridemia
iridencleisis
iridentropium
irideremia

Additional Entries

irides
iridescent vision
iridesis
iridiagnosis
iridial
iridial angle
iridian
iridic
iridic muscles
iridium
iridization
iridoavulsion
iridocapsulitis
iridocapsulotomy
iridocele
iridochoroiditis
iridocoloboma
iridoconstrictor
iridocorneal angle
iridocorneosclerectomy
iridocyclectomy
iridocyclitis
    heterochromic i.
iridocyclochoroiditis
iridocystectomy
iridodesis
iridodiagnosis
iridodialysis
iridodiastasis
iridodilator
iridodonesis
iridokeratitis
iridokinesia
iridokinesis
iridokinetic
iridoleptynsis
iridology
iridolysis

iridomalacia
iridomesodialysis
iridomotor
iridoncus
iridoparalysis
iridopathy
iridoperiphakitis
iridoplegia
    accommodation i.
    complete i.
    reflex i.
    sympathetic i.
iridoptosis
iridopupillary
iridorhexis
iridoschisis
iridosclerotomy
iridosteresis
iridotasis
iridotomy
iris
    bombe, i.
    Florentine i.
    tremulous i.
    umbrella i.
iris contraction reflex
Iri-Sol
irisopsia
iritic
iritis
    diabetic i.
    follicular i.
    gouty i.
    plastic i.
    purulent i.
    serous i.
    spongy i.
    sympathetic i.

Additional Entries

iritis *(continued)*
    uratic i.
iritoectomy
iritomy
IRMA (intraretinal microvascular abnormalities)
irradiation cataract
irregular astigmatism
irrigator
    Bishop-Harmon i.
Irvine-Gass syndrome
Irvine operation
ischemia
    i. retinae
iseikonic lens
Ishihara color test
island defects
Ismotic
isofurophate ophthalmic solution
iso-iconia
iso-iconic
isomerase
    retinal i.
    retinene i.
isometropia
isopia
isoproterenol
isopter
Isopto Atropine
Isopto Carbachol
Isopto Carpine
Isopto Cetamide
Isopto Cetapred
Isopto Homatropine
Isopto Hyoscine
isoscope
isosorbide
Isuprel
I-Temp cautery
I-Temp disposable cauteries (CooperVision Refractive Surgery)
IV slit lamp (Marco)
Iwanoff's (Iwanow's) cysts

Additional Entries

J

J1, J2, J3, etc. (Jaeger tests)
Jackson cross cylinder
Jacob's membrane
Jacob's ulcer
Jacobson's retinitis
Jaeger hook
Jaeger keratome
Jaeger lid plate
Jaeger retractor
Jaeger test type
Jaesche-Arlt operation
Jaime operation
Jameson muscle hook
Jameson operation
Jansky-Bielshowsky syndrome
Javal's ophthalmometer
jaw winking
jaw-winking syndrome
Jenning's test
Jensen choroiditis
Jensen operation
Jensen retinitis
J-Flex posterior chamber lens
J loop posterior chamber lens
Johnson knife
Johnson operation
Johnson-Tooke knife
Jones operation
Jones Pyrex tube
Jordan implant
junction
    sclerocorneal j.
juvenile cataract
juvenile developmental cataract
juvenile glaucoma
juvenile reflex
JXG (juvenile xanthogranuloma)

Additional Entries

_____
_____
_____
_____
_____
_____
_____
_____
_____
_____
_____
_____
_____
_____
_____
_____
_____
_____
_____
_____

Additional Entries

K

keratitis
- acne rosacea k.
- actinic k.
- aerosol k.
- alphabet k.
- arborescens, k.
- artificial silk k.
- bandelette, k.
- band-shaped k.
- bank k.
- bullosa, k.
- deep k.
- dendriform k.
- dendritic k.
- desiccation k.
- Dimmer's k.
- disciform k.
- disciformis, k.
- exposure k.
- fascicular k.
- filamentary k.
- filamentosa, k.
- furrow k.
- herpetic k.
- hypopyon k.
- interstitial k.
- lagophthalmic k.
- lattice k.
- marginal k.
- metaherpetic k.
- mycotic k.
- neuroparalytic k.
- neurotrophic k.
- nummularis, k.
- parenchymatous k.

keratitis *(continued)*
- petrificans, k.
- phlyctenular k.
- profunda, k.
- punctate k.
- reaper's k.
- reticular k.
- ribbon-like k.
- rosacea k.
- sclerosing k.
- scrofulus k.
- secondary k.
- serpiginous k.
- sicca, k.
- silk k.
- striate k.
- suppurative k.
- trachomatous k.
- trophic k.
- vascular k.
- vesicular k.
- xerotic k.
- zonular k.

keratocele
keratocentesis
keratoconjunctivitis
- epidemic k.
- epizootic k.
- flash k.
- phlyctenular k.
- shipyard k.
- sicca, k.
- viral k.

keratoconjunctivitis sicca
keratoconus

Additional Entries

keratoconus soft lens (Flexlens)
keratocyte
keratoderma
keratodermatocele
keratoectasia
keratoglobus
keratohelcosis
keratohemia
keratoid
keratoiditis
keratoiridocyclitis
keratoiridoscope
keratoiritis
keratoleptynsis
keratoleukoma
Keratolux internal fixation device (Carl Zeiss)
keratomalacia
keratome
    Jaeger k.
keratometer
keratometer I (Marco)
keratometric
keratometry
keratomileusis
keratomycosis
keratonosus
keratonyxis
keratopathy
    band k.
    band-shaped k.
keratoplasty
    optic k.
    tectonic k.
keratoprosthesis
keratorhexis
keratoscleritis
keratoscope

keratoscopy
keratotome
keratotomy
    delimiting k.
keratotorus
kerectasis
kerectomy
keroid
Kerrison forceps
Kestenbaum rule
Key operation
keyhole pupil
Keystone ocular telebinocular
Keystone ophthalmic telebinocular (Keystone View)
Keystone Professional Performance Test Set (Keystone View)
Keystone View
Keystone View stereopsis test
Kiloh-Nevin syndrome
kinescope
kinetic perimeters
kinetic perimetry
kinetic strabismus
King operation
King orbital implant
Kirby cataract extraction
Kirby forceps
Kirby intracapsular lens loop
Kirby intracapsular lens spoon
Kirby iris forceps
Kirby iris spatula
Kirby knife
Kirby lens dislocator
Kirby retractor
Klein keratoscope
Klieg eye

Additional Entries

Klippel-Fiel syndrome
Kloti vitreous cutter
KM-800 automatic keratometer (Marco)
Knapp cataract knife
Knapp flap operation
Knapp-Imre lid operation
Knapp iris scissors
Knapp iris spatula and hooks
Knapp lid operation
Knapp needle
Knapp pterygium operation
Knapp's forceps
Knapp's law
Knapp's operation
Knapp's streaks
Knapp-Wheeler-Reese operation
Knie's sign
knife
    Alcon Surgical k.
    Bard-Parker k.
    Beard k.
    Beaver k.
    Beer k.
    Berens k.
    Deutschman cataract k.
    Elschnig cataract k.
    Gill k.
    Goldman serrated k.
    Graefe cataract (von Graefe) k.
    Green cataract k.
    Johnson k.
    Johnson-Tooke k.
    Keeler k.
    Kirby k.
    Knapp cataract k.
    Lowell k.

knife *(continued)*
    McPherson-Ziegler k.
    McReynolds k.
    Paton k.
    Paufique k.
    Sharpoint k.
    Sichel k.
    Smith k.
    Smith-Fisher k.
    Tooke k.
    von Graefe k.
    Wheeler k.
    Ziegler k.
knife needle
Knolle intraocular lens
Koby's cataract
Koch-Weeks bacillus
Kocher's sign
Koeppe gonioscopic lens implant
Koeppe nodules
Koffler operation
KOH (potassium hydroxide)
KOI 3000X ultrasonic pachymeter (CooperVision Refractive Surgery)
KOI diamond knife (CooperVision Refractive Surgery)
KOI instrument tray
KOI sterilization tray (CooperVision Refractive Surgery)
Koteline bifocal lens
Kowa 45 deg./30 deg./20 deg. automatic fundus camera (Kowa)
Kowa automated slit lamp (Kowa)

Additional Entries

Kowa hand camera
Kowa Optimed
Kowa PRO 1/50/35/20 fundus camera
Kowa RC-2 fundus camera
Kowa RC-XV2 fundus camera
Kowa slit lamp
Koyter's muscle
KP (keratic precipitates)
Krabbe's disease
Kratz lens
Kratz scratcher
Kratz-Johnson intraocular lens
Kraupa operation
Krause's glands
K-readings
Kreiker blepharochalasis
Krieberg operation
Krimsky test
Kronfeld retractor
Kronlein-Berke operation
Krukenberg pigment spindle
Krupin valve
Krwawicz cataract extractor
Kryptok bifocal lens
Kryptok bifocals lens implant
Kufs' disease
Kuhnt dacryostomy
Kuhnt eyelid operation
Kuhnt-Junius disease
Kuhnt tarsectomy
Kuhnt's illusion
Kuhnt's intermediary tissue
Kuhnt's postcentral vein
Kuhnt-Helmbold operation
Kuhnt-Junius disease
Kuhnt-Szymanowski eyelid operation
Kuhnt-Thorpe operation
Kulvin-Kalt forceps
kuttarosome
Kwito operation
kyanophane

Additional Entries

L

Lacarrere operation
lacerate foramen, anterior
lacquer cracks
Lacril
Lacri-Lube S.O.P.
lacrimal
lacrimal abscess
lacrimal apparatus
lacrimal bay
lacrimal canal
lacrimal crest, anterior
lacrimal crest, posterior
lacrimal duct
lacrimal fistula
lacrimal fossa
lacrimal gland
lacrimal glands, accessory
lacrimal groove
lacrimal lake
lacrimal notch of maxilla
lacrimal papilla
lacrimal point
lacrimal probe
lacrimal reflex
lacrimal sac
lacrimal sulcus of lacrimal bone
lacrimal sulcus of maxilla
lacrimal vein
lacrimalis
    l. lamina
    l. lateral canthus
    l. levator palpebrae
lacrimation
lacrimoconchal suture
lacrimomaxillary suture
lacrimonasal duct
lacrimoturbinal suture
Lacrisert
lacteal cataract
lacus
    l. lacrimalis
Lagleyze eyelid operation
Lagleyze-Trantas operation
lagophthalmic keratitis
lagophthalmos
Lagrange modification of Arruga operation
Lagrange modification of Berens operation
Lagrange operation
laissez-faire lid operation
lake
    lacrimal l.
Lambert forceps
lamellar cataract
lamellar corneal graft
lamellar developmental cataract
lamellar graft
lamellar keratoplasty
lamina
    anterior limiting l.
    basal l. of ciliary body
    basal l. of choroid
    Bowman's l.
    episcleral l.
    limiting l., anterior
    limiting l., posterior
    suprachoroid l.
lamp
    Birch-Hirschfeld l.

Additional Entries

lamp *(continued)*
    Eldridge-Green l.
    Gullstrand's slit l.
    Haag-Streit slit l.
    Hague cataract l.
    Rodenstock slit l.
    Zeiss slit l.
Lancaster lid speculum
Lancaster operation
Lancaster-Regan dial #1
Lancaster-Regan dial #2
Lanchner operation
Landegger orbital implant
Landolt's bodies
Landolt's operation
Landstrom's muscle
Langenbeck operation
lantern test
larval conjunctivitis
LASAG Microruptor (SITE)
LASAG Topaz Nd:YAG Laser (SITE)
laser (argon/YAG)
    Allergan Humphrey l.
    Biophysic Medical l.
    Carl Zeiss l.
    CILCO l.
    Coherent Medical l.
    CooperVision l.
    CooperVision Surgical l.
    Lasertek l.
    Ophthalas l.
    SITE l.
Laserflex intraocular lens
latent hyperopia
latent strabismus
lateral angle of eye
lateral canthus
lateral commissure of eyelid
lateral hemianopia
lateral medullary syndrome
lateral orbital tubercle
lateral palpebral tubercle
lateral phoria
lateral rectus muscle
lattice degeneration of retina
lattice dystrophy of cornea
lattice keratitis
Laurence-Moon-Biedl syndrome
law
    Desmarres' l.
    Donder's l.
    Giraud-Teulon l.
    Gullstrand's l.
    Hering's l.
    Horner's l.
    Knapp's l.
    Listing's l.
    Wundt-Lamansky l.
Lawford's syndrome
layer
    bacillary l.
    Bowman's l.
    Chievitz l.
    columnar l.
    ganglion cell l.
    ganglionic l. of optic nerve
    ganglionic l. of retina
    Henle's fiber l.
    molecular l., inner
    molecular l., outer
    neuroepithelial l. of retina
    nuclear l., inner
    nuclear l., outer
    pigmented l. of ciliary body

Additional Entries

layer *(continued)*
    pigmented l. of eyeball
    pigmented l. of iris
    pigmented l. of retina
    plexiform l's.
    rods and cones, l. of
lazy eye
LC-65 daily contact lens cleaner (Allergan)
Leahey operation
Lebensohn chart
Leber's congenital amaurosis
Leber's disease
Leber's optic atrophy
Lederle Laboratories
Lederle Parenterals
Leeming Division
legal blindness
lemnisci
lemniscus
    optic l.
Lemoine orbital implant
lens
    Accugel l.
    Accugel Thin l.
    acrylic l.
    adherent l.
    American IOL International l.
    American Medical Optics intraocular l.
    Amsof l.
    Amsofthin l.
    Aosoft l.
    aplanatic l.
    apochromatic l.
    Aquaflex l.
    Aquasight l.

lens *(continued)*
    bandage l.
    baseball l.
    biconcave l.
    biconvex l.
    bicylindrical l.
    bifocal l.
    Binkhorst 2 loop l.
    Binkhorst 4 loop l.
    Binkhorst-Fyodorov l.
    Bi-Soft l.
    bispherical l.
    bitoric contact l.
    Brucke l.
    cataract l.
    Choyce l.
    Cibasoft low plus l.
    Cibasoft minus l.
    Cibathin l.
    CILCO intraocular l.
    Coburn/Rayner intraocular l.
    compound l.
    concave l.
    concavoconcave l.
    concavoconvex l.
    contact l.
    converging l.
    convex l.
    convexoconcave l.
    CooperVision IOL l.
    Copeland Intralenses intraocular l.
    Coquille plano l.
    Crookes' l.
    crossed l.
    crystalline l.
    CSI daily wear l.
    CSI T extended wear l.

Additional Entries

lens *(continued)*
- CustomEyes l.
- cylindrical l.
- decentered l.
- Deltacon Standard l.
- deltafilcon XT l.
- dispersing l.
- DuraSoft 2 l.
- DuraSoft 3 l.
- Flexlens l.
- Frelex l.
- Genesis 4 l.
- Hydracon l.
- Hydracon toric l.
- Hydrocurve extended wear soft l.
- Hydron Custom toric l.
- Hydron Mini l.
- Hydron spincast l.
- Hydron X-70 l.
- Hydron Zero 4 l.
- Hydron Zero 4F l.
- Hydron Zero 6 l.
- Hydron Zero T l.
- Hydron Z plus l.
- HydroSight l.
- HydroSight Thin l.
- immersion l.
- Intermedics intraocular l.
- IOLAB intraocular l.
- IOPTEX intraocular l.
- iseikonic l.
- McGhan/3M intraocular l.
- meniscus l.
- meter l.
- Metro 55 l.
- Metrosoft II l.
- minus l.

lens *(continued)*
- omnifocal l.
- Optical Radiation intraocular l.
- orthoscopic l.
- PDC-70 l.
- periscopic l.
- Permaflex HGP l.
- Permaflex-Thin l.
- Permaflex-Thin 43 l.
- Permalens l.
- Permalens extended wear soft l.
- Permalens-Aphakic l.
- Pharmacia Ophthalmics intraocular l.
- planoconcave l.
- planoconvex l.
- plus l.
- Precision Cosmet intraocular l.
- prosthetic l.
- punktal l.
- retroscopic l.
- Sauflon extended wearsoft l.
- Sauflon 70 l.
- Sofact II l.
- Sof-form II l.
- Softcon l.
- Soft-Mate l.
- Soft-Mate II l.
- Soft Mate B l.
- Soft Mate DW l.
- Soft Mate EW l.
- spherical l.
- Storz intraocular l.
- Surgidev intraocular l.

Additional Entries

lens *(continued)*
    Synsoft bifocal l.
    Torisoft l.
    Tresoft l.
    trial l.
    trifocal l.
    Vistakon l.
    Vistamarc l.
    Wesley Jessen l.
Lens Clear
lens dislocation
Lens Fresh
lens glide
lens nucleus
Lens Plus
lens rudiment
lens star
lens vesicle
lens whorl
lens zonule
Lensine
LensKeeper
LensKeeper contact lens carrying case (Allergan)
Lens-Mate
lensometer
    Allergan Humphrey l.
    Carl Zeiss l.
    Coburn l.
    Marco l.
    Reichert l.
    Topcon l.
Lensrins
Lensventory contact lens organizer cabinets (VanIderstine Designs)
Lens-Wet
lentectomize
lentectomy
lenticonus
lenticula
lenticular
lenticular astigmatism
lenticular body
lenticular cataract
lenticular degeneration
lenticular fossa
lenticular glaucoma
lenticular nucleus
lenticulo-optic
lenticulostriate
lenticulothalamic
lentiform
lentiform nucleus
lentiglobus
lentitis
lentoptosis
lesser ring of iris
Lester Jones operation
letter blindness
leukemic retinitis
leukemic retinopathy
leukocoria
leukoma
    l. adhaerens
leukoscope
levator palpebrae superioris
Levitt eye implant
levoduction
levoversion
Lexer operation
LGB (lateral geniculate body)
LGN (lateral geniculate nucleus)
LHT (left hypertropia)
Lichtenberg trephine
lid lag

Additional Entries

lid margin
lid reflex
lidofilcon
Liebreich's symptom
ligament
    Hueck's l.
    hyaloideocapsular l.
    suspensory l.
ligamenta
    l. pectinatum anguli iridocornealis
    l. pectinatum iridis
light
    difference, l.
    idioretinal l.
    intrinsic l.
light adaptation
light coagulation
light minimum
light perception
light projection
light reflex
light sensitivity (photophobia)
light-adapted eye
light-near dissociation
lightning cataract
lightning degenerative cataract
Lignac-Fanconi syndrome
limbus
    conjunctivae, ll.
    cornea, l. of
    luteus retinae, ll.
    palpebrales anteriores, ll.
    palpebrales posteriores, ll.
limiting lamina, anterior
limiting lamina, posterior
limulus lysate test
Lincoff implant
Lincoff operation
Lindau-von Hippel disease
Linde cryogenic probe
Lindner operation
Lindner sclerotomy
Lindsay operation
line
    atropic l.
    fixation, l. of
    Morgan's l.
    sight, l. of
    triradiate l's
    visual l.
    Zollner's l.
linea
    l. visus
lines
    Fraunhofer's l's
lipemia
    l. retinalis
lipoma
lippa
lippitude
Lipschutz's bodies
Liquifilm
Liquifilm Tears
Lister forceps
Listing's law
Listing's plane
lithiasis
    l. conjunctivae
LKP (lamellar keratoplasty)
LM850 automatic lensmeter
local tic
localizer
    Berman l.
    Roper-Hall l.
    Wildgen-Reck l.

Additional Entries

logadectomy
logaditis
Lohlein operation
Londermann corneal trephine
long root of ciliary ganglion
long sight
long-scale contrast
loop
    Arlt l.
    Kirby intracapsular lens l.
    Meyer l.
    New Orleans lens l.
loops of Axenfeld
Lopez-Enriquez scleral trephine
Lordan forceps
Louis-Bar syndrome
loupe
Lovac fundus contact lens implant
Lovac six mirror gonioscopic lens implant
low contrast
Lowe's ring
Lowe's syndrome
Lowell knife
Lowenstein operation
lower hemianopia
lower retina
Lowe-Terry-Machlachan syndrome
L proj (light projection)
LP (light perception and light projection)
LP/Proj. (light perception with projection)
LR (lateral rectus)
Lubrifair
lucite sphere orbital implant
luminance
Lundsgaard-Burch rasp
luxation
Lyda Ivalon-Lucite orbital implant
lymphoma
lymphomatosis
    ocular l.
lysozyme
Lyteers

Additional Entries

Additional Entries

M

Machek ptosis operation
Machek-Blaskovics operation
Machek-Gifford operation
Machemer vitreous cutter
MacKay-Marg electronic tonometer
Mack-Brunswick operation
macroblepharia
macrocornea
macrophthalmia
macrophthalmos
macropia
macropsia
macula
    m. corneae
    m., false
    m. flava retinae
    m. lutea retinae
    m. retinae
maculae
macular
macular arteriole, inferior
macular arteriole, superior
macular corneal dystrophy
macular degeneration
macular pucker
macular sparing
macular splitting
macular star
macular stereopsis
macular suppression
macular venule, inferior
macular venule, superior
maculate
macule
maculocerebral
Maddos prism
Maddox rod
Maddox rod test
Maddox wing
Magitot keratoplasty
magnet
    Gruning's m.
    Haab's m.
    Hirschberg's m.
magnet operation
magnification
Magnus operation
Maguire-Harvey vitreous cutter
main fibers
Majewski operation
Maladie de Greffe operation
Malbec operation
Malbran operation
malignant exophthalmos
malignant glaucoma
malignant myopia
malprojection
mandibulofacial dysostosis
mandibulo-oculofacial dyscephaly
Manhattan eye forceps
manifest deviation
manifest hyperopia
manifest strabismus
mannitol
Mann's sign
manoptoscope
Manz's glands
Marchesani's syndrome
Marco chart projector

Additional Entries

Marco Equipment
Marco lensometer
Marco LM850 automatic lensmeter
Marco MTL trial frame
Marco perimeter
Marco radiusgauge
Marco refractor
Marco RT-1 refractor
Marco SurgiScope
Marco IIB slit lamp
Marco III slit lamp
Marco IV slit lamp
Marco V slit lamp
Marco V-G slit lamp
Marcus Gunn pupillary sign
Marcus Gunn syndrome
margin
    ciliary m. of iris
    free m. of eyelid
    infraorbital m. of maxilla
    infraorbital m. of orbit
    pupillary m. of iris
    supraorbital m. of orbit
marginal blepharitis
marginal catarrhal ulcer
marginal keratitis
marginal myotomy
marginoplasty
margo
    m. ciliaris iridis
    m. infraorbitalis orbitae
    m. lacrimalis maxillae
    m. pupillaris iridis
    m. supraorbitalis orbitae
    m. supraorbitalis ossis frontalis
Marinesco-Sjogren syndrome

Mariotte's spot
Marquez-Gomez conjunctival graft
Masselon's spectacles
Mattis scissors
Mauksch operation
Maumenee and Goldberg operation
Maumenee-Park speculum
Maunoir scissors
Max Fine forceps
Maxidex
Maxitrol
Maxwell's ring
Maxwell's spot
Mayo scissors
McCarthy's reflex
McClure scissors
McCullough forceps
McGavic operation
McGhan/3M intraocular lens
McGuire forceps
McGuire operation
McGuire scissors
McIntyre style handpiece
McKinney fixation ring
McLaughlin operation
McLean forceps
McLean operation
McLean sutures
McLean tonometer
McPherson forceps
McPherson-Vannas scissors
McPherson-Ziegler knife
McReynolds transplant of pterygium
McReynolds hook
McReynolds keratome

Additional Entries

McReynolds knife
McReynolds operation
McReynolds scissors
meatus
    m. nasi inferior
mechanical strabismus
mechanism
    oculogyric m.
Mecholyl
Medallion lens
medial angle of eye
medial arteriole of retina
medial canthus
medial commissure of eyelids
medial horn
medial palpebral ligament
medial rectus
medial venule of retina
medicamentosa conjunctivitis
medium
    dioptric mm.
    refracting mm.
Meek operation
Meesman dystrophy
megalocornea
megalophthalmos
megalopia
megalopsia
megophthalmos
meibomian glands
meibomian stye
melanin
melanocytes
melanocytoma
melanoma
melanosis
    m. oculi
    m. sclerae

Melauskas orbital implant
Melkersson's syndrome
Melkersson-Rosenthal syndrome
Meller operation
Meller retractor
membrana
    m. epipapillaris
    m. fusca
    m. granulosa externa
    m. granulosa interna
    m. hyaloidea
    m. orbitalis musculosa
    m. pupillaris
    m. vitrea
membrane
    Bowman's m.
    cyclitic m.
    Demours' m.
    Descemet's m.
    Duddell's m.
    nictitating m.
    pupillary m.
    purpurogenous m.
    Reichert's m.
    vitreous m.
    Wachendorf's m.
    Zinn's m.
membranous cataract
membranous conjunctivitis
Mendez ultrasonic cystotome
meningioma
meningococcus conjunctivitis
meniscus lens
Mentor wet field coagulator
Merck Sharp & Dohme
meridian
    m. of cornea
    m's of eyeball

Additional Entries

meridiani
meridianus
    mm. bulbi oculi
meridional
meridional amblyopia
meridional fibers of ciliary
    muscle
meropia
mesocornea
mesodermal dysgenesis
mesophryon
mesopia
mesopic
mesoretina
mesoropter
metaherpetic keratitis
metameric color
metamorphopsia
metarhodopsin
metastatic choroiditis
metastatic retinitis
methacholine
methazolamide
methicillin
method
    Crede's m.
    Cuignet's m.
    direct m.
    Hirschberg's m.
    optical density m.
Methulose
methylcellulose
methylprednisolone
Metimyd
metric ophthalmoscopy
Metro 55 contact lens, soft
Metrosoft II contact lens, soft
Meyer's loop

Meyer-Schwickerath light
    coagulation
Meyhoeffer curet
MG (Marcus Gunn pupil)
mica spectacles
Michaelson counter pressure
microaneurysm
microblepharia
microblepharism
microblepharon
microblephary
microcoria
microcornea
microgonioscope
micrometer disk
micronystagmus
Microphake cryoextractor
microphakia
microphthalmia
microphthalmoscope
microphthalmus
micropsia
microsaccades
microscope
    corneal m.
    Zeiss operating m.
microscopy
    fundus m.
microspherophakia
Microsponge
microstrabismus
migraine
    ophthalmic m.
    ophthalmoplegic m.
Mikulicz's syndrome
milia
miliary aneurysm
milky cataract

Additional Entries

Millard-Gubler syndrome
Miller-Nadler glaretester
millimicron
mind blindness
miner's nystagmus
mini-ophthalmic drape
minimum
    light m.
    visible, m.
minimum deviation
minimum visual angle
Minsky operation
Minsky intramarginal splinting
Minsky's circles
minus cyclophoria
minus cyclotropia
Miocel
Miochol
miosis
Miostat
miotic
Mira diathermy
Mira unit
Miracon
Miraflow
Mirasept
mire
mirror haploscope
mirror image
Mittendorf's dot
mixed astigmatism
mixed cataract
MK IV ophthalmoscope
MLF (medial longitudinal fasciculus)
Mobius' syndrome
modified C loop intraocular lens
modified J loop intraocular lens

Moehle forceps
molecular layer, inner
molecular layer, outer
Moll glands
Moller microscope
molluscum conjunctivitis
Monakow's syndrome
Moncrieff discission
monoblepsia
monochromasy
monochromat
monochromatic eye
monocular
monocular diplopia
monocular strabismus
monocular vision
monoculus
monodiplopia
monofixation
monolateral strabismus
monopia
moon blindness
Mooren's ulcer
Moran proptosis
Morax keratoplasty
Morax-Axenfeld's conjunctivitis
Morel-Fatio-Lalardie operation
morgagnian cataract
Morgan's line
morning ptosis
Morquio-Brailsford syndrome
Mosher operation
Mosher-Toti operation
Moss traction
Motais operation
Mot-R-Pak vitrectomy system
motor
    m. oculi

Additional Entries

motor root of ciliary ganglion
motor tic
MR (medial rectus)
MTL trial frame
mucoitin sulfate
mucoitin-sulfuric acid
mucormycosis
mucotome
Mueller shield
Mueller trephine
Mulberger orbital implant
Mules implant
Mules operation
Muller's fibers
Muller's muscle
Muller's operation
multifocal lens
Multilux
multiple vision
Munson's sign
mural cells
Murine Plus
Murine Regular
Muro 128
Muro Tears
Muro's Opcon
Muro's Opcon-A
Murocel
Murocoll 2
muscae volitantes
muscle
    Bowman's m.
    Brucke's m.
    ciliary m.
    iridic m's
    Koyter's m.
    Landstrom's m.
    Muller's m.

muscle *(continued)*
    oblique m. of eyeball, inferior
    oblique m. of eyeball, superior
    orbicular m. of eye
    Riolan's m.
    Rouget's m.
    sphincter m. of pupil
    yoked m's
muscle cone
muscle hook
muscular asthenopia
muscular fasciae of eye
muscular funnel
muscular strabismus
musculi
    m. bulbi
    m. ciliaris
    m. corrugator supercilii
    m. depressor supercilii
    m. dilator pupillae
    m. levator palpebrae superioris
    m. obliquus inferior bulbi
    m. obliquus inferior oculi
    m. obliquus superior bulbi
    m. obliquus superior oculi
    m. oculi
    m. orbicularis
    m. orbicularis oculi
    m. orbitalis
    m. procerus
    m. rectus inferior bulbi
    m. rectus inferior oculi
    m. rectus lateralis bulbi
    m. rectus lateralis oculi
    m. rectus medialis bulbi

Additional Entries

musculi *(continued)*
    m. rectus medialis oculi
    m. rectus superior bulbi
    m. rectus superior oculi
    m. sphincter pupillae
    m. tarsalis inferior
    m. tarsalis superior
mushroom corneal graft
Mustarde graft
MVS XIV surgical system
MVS XII surgical system
MVS XX surgical system
myasthenia gravis
mycotic keratitis
Mydfrin
Mydrapred
Mydriacyl
Mydriafair
mydriasis
    alternating m.
    bounding m.
    paralytic m.
    spasmodic m.
    spastic m.
    spinal m.
    springing m.
mydriatic
myectomy of ocular muscle

myiocephalon
myiocephalum
myiodesopsia
myodiopter
Myodisc
myokymia
myopathy
    ocular m.
myope
myopia
    axial m.
    chromic m.
    curvature m.
    index m.
    malignant m.
    pernicious m.
    prodromal m.
    progressive m.
    refractive m.
myopic
myopic astigmatism
myopic astigmatism, compound
myopic astigmatism, simple
myopic conus
myopic crescent
myopic reflex
myotomy of ocular muscle

Additional Entries

Additional Entries

N

N (nasal)
Nafazair
Nafazair A
Naffziger operation
Nagel's test
Nairobi eye
Nanolas Nd:YAG laser system (Biophysic Medical)
nanometer
nanophthalmos
naphazoline hydrochloride
Naphcon
Naphcon Forte
Naphcon-A
naphthalinic cataract
narrow-angle glaucoma
nasal arteriole of retina, inferior
nasal arteriole of retina, superior
nasal canal
nasal duct
nasal hemianopia
nasal retina
nasal venule of retina, inferior
nasal venule of retina, superior
nasociliary
nasociliary neuralgia
nasolacrimal
nasolacrimal canal
nasolacrimal duct
Natacyn
natamycin
NCT II
near point
near point of convergence
near point, absolute
near point, relative
near-sight
nearsighted
nearsightedness
near vision
nebula
necroticans infectiosus conjunctivitis
necrotizing papillitis
needle
    Bowman cataract n.
    Daily cataract n.
    Kelman n.
    knife n.
    Ziegler n.
needle holder
    Castroviejo n.h.
    Castroviejo-Kalt n.h.
    Kalt n.h.
needling of lens
negative accommodation
negative convergence
negative cyclophoria
negative cyclotropia
negative eyepiece
negative image
negative scotoma
negative vertical divergence
Neher operation
Nehra-Mack ptosis operation
Neo Cortef
Neo Dexair
NeoDecadron

Additional Entries

neomycin sulfate, polymyxin B
  sulfate and gramicidin
  ophthalmic
  solution
Neosporin
Neosynephrine
Neo-Tears
neovascular glaucoma
nephelopia
Neptazane
nerve
  ciliary n's, long
  ciliary n's, short
  infraorbital n.
  ophthalmic n.
  optic n.
nervi
  n. abducens
  n. ciliares breves
  n. ciliares longi
  n. infraorbitalis
  n. lacrimalis
  n. maxillaris
  n. nasociliaris
  n. oculomotorius
  n. ophthalmicus
  n. opticus
  n. supraorbitalis
  n. trigeminus
  n. trochlearis
  n. zygomaticus
nervous asthenopia
Nettleship iris repositor
network
  peritarsal n.
neuralgia
  nasociliary n.
  supraorbital n.

neurectomy
  opticociliary n.
neuritis
  optic n.
  orbital optic n.
  postocular n.
  retrobulbar n.
neurochorioretinitis
neurochoroiditis
neurodealgia
neurodeatrophia
neuroepithelial layer of retina
neuromyelitis
  n. optica
neuron
  Golgi type I n's
  Golgi type II n's
neuro-ophthalmology
neuroparalytic keratitis
neuroretinitis
neuroretinopathy
  hypertensive n.
neurospongium
neurotrophic keratitis
neutrality
New Orleans loop
nictitating membrane
Nida operation
Niemann-Pick disease
night blindness
night sight
night vision
nigroid body
Nikon external camera
niphablepsia
niphotyphlosis
nitronaphthalene
Nizetic operation

Additional Entries

NLP (no light perception)
Nocito eye implant
nocturnal amblyopia
nodal point
nodular conjunctivitis
nodule
    Busacca n's
    lentiform n.
nodulus
    nn. lymphatici conjunctivales
Nokrome bifocal lens
nonaccommodative esotropia
noncomitant heterotropia
noncomitant strabismus
nonconcomitant strabismus
noncongestive glaucoma
Non-Contact tonometer (NCT)
Non-Contact II tonometer (Reichert)
nongranulomatous uveitis
nonparalytic strabismus
Norman-Wood syndrome
Normol
Norrie's disease
notch
    lacrimal n. of maxilla
note blindness
Nova Curve laser lens optic
Nova Flex PMMA haptics
Nova Curve broad C-loop posterior chamber lens
Nova Curve Omnicurve
Noyes scissors

NPA (near point of accommodation)
NPC (near point of convergence)
nuclear cataract
nuclear developmental cataract
nuclear layer, inner
nuclear layer, outer
nuclear ophthalmoplegia
nucleus
    accessory n.
    lenticular n.
    lentiform n.
    pretectal n.
Nugent hook
Nugent soft cataract aspirator
null point
nyctalope
nyctalopia
nystagmic
nystagmiform
nystagmograph
nystagmoid
nystagmus
    caloric n.
    endpoint n.
    labyrinthine n.
    latent n.
    miner's n.
    optokinetic n.
    paretic n.
    pendular n.
    rotatory n.
    vestibular n.
nystagmus-myoclonus

Additional Entries

Additional Entries

O

obcecation
object blindness
oblique astigmatism
oblique muscle of eyeball, inferior
oblique muscle of eyeball, superior
O'Brien akinesia
O'Brien block
O'Brien cataract
O'Brien forceps
Obrite
obstructive glaucoma
OC-20 automated ophthalmic chairs (Topcon Instrument)
occipital cortex
occipitothalamic radiation
occluder
occlusion
O'Connor forceps
O'Connor operation
O'Connor-Peter operation
Octopus
Ocu-Caine
Ocu-Carpine
Ocu-Chlor
Ocu-Cort
Ocu-Dex
Ocugestrin
ocular
ocular albinism
ocular angle
ocular bobbing
ocular cone
ocular crisis

ocular cup
ocular dominance
ocular dysmetria
ocular histoplasmosis
ocular humor
ocular hypertelorism
ocular hypotelorism
ocular image
ocular lymphomatosis
ocular myoclonus
ocular myopathy
ocular paralysis
ocular pemphigus
ocular phthisis
ocular prosthesis
ocular refraction
ocular spectrum
ocular torticollis
ocular vesicle
oculentum
oculi
oculi uterque (OU)
oculist
oculistics
oculoauricular dysplasia
oculoauriculovertebral dysplasia
oculocephalogyric
oculocephalogyric reflex
oculocerebro-vasculometer (Topcon Instrument)
oculocutaneous
oculodentodigital dysplasia
oculofacial
oculogyration
oculogyria

Additional Entries

_____
_____
_____
_____
_____

oculogyric
oculogyric crisis
oculogyric mechanism
oculometroscope
oculomotor
oculomotor (III) nerve
oculomotor root of ciliary
   ganglion
oculomotorius
oculomycosis
oculonasal
Ocu-Lone-C
oculopathy
oculopharyngeal reflex
oculopupillary
oculopupillary reflex
oculoreaction
oculosensory cell reflex
oculospinal
Ocu-Lube
oculus
   o. dexter (OD)
   o. sinister (OS)
Ocumed
Ocu-Mycin
Ocu-Pentolate
Ocu-Phrin
Ocu-Pred
Ocu-Pred A
Ocu-Pred Forte
Ocusert Pilo-20
Ocusert Pilo-40
Ocu-Sol
Ocu-Spor-B
Ocu-Spor-G
Ocu-Sul-10
Ocu-Sul-15
Ocu-Sul-30

Ocu-Tears
ocutome
Ocutricin
Ocutricin HC
Ocu-Trol
Ocu-Tropic
Ocu-Tropine
Ocu-Zoline
OCVM system
   oculocerebro-vasculometer
   (Digilab)
OD (oculus dexter - right eye)
ODN (ophthalmodynamometry)
Ogston-Luc operation
Oguchi's disease
OHT (ocular hypertensive)
ointment
   sodium sulfacetamide
      ophthalmic o.
OKN (optokinetic nystagmus)
old sight
Olympus GRC-WT fundus
   camera
O'Malley self-adhering lens
   implants
O'Malley-Heintz vitreous cutter
O'Malley-Heintz cutter
OM 200 microscope (Marco)
OM 2000 operation microscope
   (Marco)
OM-4 ophthalmometer (Topcon
   Instrument)
Onchocerca
onchocerciasis
onchocercosis
one-snip punctum
One solution
open-angle glaucoma

Additional Entries

opening
    orbital o.
open-sky cryoextraction
operations
    Adams
    Adler
    Agnew
    Allen
    Allport
    Alsus-Knapp
    Alvis
    Ammon
    Amsler
    Anagnostakis
      (Hotz-Anagnostakis)
    Angelucci
    annular corneal graft
    Argyll Robertson
    Arion
    Arlt
    Arlt-Jaesche
    Arrowhead
      (Wicherkiewicz)
    Arruga
    Arruga-Berens
    Badal's
    Bangerter
    Bardelli
    Barkan
    Barkan-Cordes
    Barraquer
    Barrie Jones
    Beard-Cut
    Beer's
    Benedict
    Berens
    Berens-Smith
    Berke

operations *(continued)*
    Berke-Motais
    Bethke
    Bielschowsky
    Birch-Hirschfeld
    Blair
    Blasius
    Blaskovics
    Blaskovics-Berke
    Bohm's
    Bonaccolto-Flieringa
    Bonnett
    Bonzel
    Borthen
    Bossalino
    Bowman
    Boyd
    Brailey
    Bridge
    Briggs
    Bromley
    Bronson
    Budinger
    Burch
    Burow
    Buzzi
    Byron Smith
    Cairns
    Caldwell-Luc
    Calhoun-Hagler
    Callahan
    Campodonico
    Carter
    Casanellas
    Casey
    Castroviejo
    Castroviejo-Scheie
    cataract gonfle

Additional Entries

operations *(continued)*
    cautery
    Celsus
    Celsus-Hotz
    cerclage
    Chandler
    Chandler-Verhoeff
    Cibis
    Cleasby
    Comberg
    Conrad
    Cooper
    Crawford
    Crescent
    Critchett
    Crock
    cryotherapy
    Csapody
    Cusick
    Cusick-Sarrail
    Custodis
    Cutler
    Cutler-Beard
    cyclodiathermy
    Czermak
    D'ombrain
    dacryoadenectomy
    dacryocystectomy
    dacryocystostomy
    dacryocystorhinostomy
    dacryocystotomy
    Daily
    Dalgleish
    Daviel
    decompression of orbit
    de Grandmont
    Deiter's
    DeKlair

operations *(continued)*
    de Lapersonne
    Derby
    Desmarres
    deWecker
    Dianoux
    diathermy
    Dickey
    Dickey-Fox
    Dickson Wright
    Dieffenbach
    dilation of punctum
    discission of lens
    drainage of lacrimal gland
    drainage of lacrimal sac
    Duke-Elder
    Dunnington
    Dupuy-Dutemps
    Durr
    Duverger-Velter
    Elliot
    Elschnig
    encirclement of the globe
    encircling for scleral buckle
    enucleation of eyeball
    equilibrating
    Erbakan
    Escapini
    Esser
    Everbusch
    evisceration
    Ewing
    excision of lacrimal gland
    excision of lacrimal sac
    exenteration of orbital contents
    extracapsular extraction of cataract

Additional Entries

operations *(continued)*
- Fanta
- Fasanella-Servat
- Fergus
- Filatov
- Filatov-Marzinkowsky
- filtering
- Fink
- Flajani
- fluorescence retinal photography
- Fould
- Fox
- Franceschetti
- Fricke
- Friede
- Friedenwald
- Friedenwald-Guyton
- Frost-Lang
- Fuchs
- Fukala
- Gaillard
- Gayet
- Georgariou
- Gifford
- Gillies
- Girard
- Goldmann-Larsson
- Gomez-Marquez
- Gonin
- goniotomy
- Gradle
- Graefe
- graft of cornea
- Greaves
- Grimsdale
- Grossmann
- Gutzeit

operations *(continued)*
- Guyton
- Halpin
- Harman
- Harms-Dannheim
- Hasner
- Heine
- Heisrath
- Hess
- Hiff
- Hippel
- Hogan
- Holth
- Horay
- Horvath
- Hotz
- Hotz-Anagnostakis
- Hughes
- Hunt-Transley
- Iliff
- Iliff-Haus
- Imre
- indentation
- intracapsular extraction of cataract
- iridectomy
- iridencleisis
- iridodialysis
- iridotasis
- iridotomy
- Irvine
- Jaesche
- Jaesche-Arlt
- Jaime
- Jameson
- Jensen
- Johnson
- Jones

Additional Entries

operations *(continued)*
    Katzin
    Kelman
    keratectomy
    keratocentesis
    keratomileusis
    keratoplasty
    keratotomy, delimiting
    Key
    King
    Kirby
    Knapp
    Knapp-Imre
    Knapp-Wheeler-Reese
    Koffler
    Kraupa
    Kreiker
    Krieberg
    Kronlein
    Kronlein-Berke
    Kuhnt
    Kuhnt-Helmbold
    Kuhnt-Szymanowski
    Kuhnt-Thorpe
    Kwito
    Lacarrere
    Lagleyze
    Lagleyze-Trantas
    Lagrange
    laissez-faire
    Lancaster
    Lanchner
    Landolt
    Langenbeck
    laser
    Leahy
    Lester Jones
    Lexer

operations *(continued)*
    light
    Lincoff
    Lindner
    Lindsay Rea
    Lohlein
    Londermann
    Lopez-Enriquez
    Lowenstein
    Machek
    Machek-Blaskovics
    Machek-Gifford
    Mack-Brunswick
    Magitot
    magnet
    Magnus
    Majewski
    Maladie de Greffe
    Malbec
    Malbran
    Marquez-Gomez
    Mauksch
    Maumenee and Goldberg
    McGavic
    McGuire
    McLaughlin
    McLean
    McReynolds
    Meek
    Meller
    Meyer-Schwickerath
    Michaelson
    Minsky
    Moncrieff
    Moran
    Morax
    Morel-Fatio-Lalardie
    Mosher-Toti

Additional Entries

operations *(continued)*
- Moss
- Motais
- Mueller
- Mules
- Muller
- Mustarde
- myectomy
- myotomy
- Naffziger
- needling of lens
- Neher
- Nehra-Mack
- Nida
- Nizetic
- O'Connor
- O'Connor-Peter
- Ogston-Luc
- one-snip punctum
- open-sky cryoextraction
- optical iridectomy
- orbital implant
- Pagenstecher
- Panas
- pars plana
- pattern cut corneal graft
- Paufique
- peripheral iridectomy
- Peter
- Pico
- plastic
- platinum chloride tattoo
- plombage
- pocket
- Polyak
- Poulard
- Poulard-Pochissov
- Power

operations *(continued)*
- Preziosi
- probing of lacrimonasal duct
- pupil-to-root iridectomy
- Putenney
- Quaglino
- Raverdino
- Ray-Brunswick-Mack
- Ray-McLean
- reattachment of choroid
- reattachment of retina
- recession of ocular muscle
- Redmond Smith
- Reese
- Reese-Cleasby
- Reese-Jones-Cooper
- removal of foreign body
- Rochat
- Rosenburg
- Rosengren
- Rovda Y-V
- Rowbotham
- Rowinski
- Rubbrecht
- Ruedemann
- Rycroft
- Saemisch
- Safar
- Sanders
- Sato
- Savin
- Sayoc
- Scheie
- Schepens
- Schimek
- Schirmer
- Schmalz

Additional Entries

operations *(continued)*
    scleral fistula
    scleral shortening
    sclerectomy
    scleroplasty
    sclerotomy
    sector iridectomy
    Selinger
    Shaffer
    Shugrue
    Sichi
    Silva-Costa
    Silver-Hildreth
    slant
    Smith
    Snellen
    Soria
    Soriano
    Sourdille
    Spaeth
    Speas
    Spencer-Watson
    splitting of lacrimal papilla
    Stallard
    Stallard-Liegard
    step graft
    Stock
    Stocker
    Straith
    Strampelli-Valvo
    Streatfield
    Streatfield-Fox
    Streatfield-Snellen
    Suarez-Villafranca
    Summerskill
    suture of cornea
    suture of eyeball
    suture of iris

operations *(continued)*
    suture of sclera
    Szymanowski
    Szymanowski-Kuhnt
    Tansley
    Tasia
    tattoo of cornea
    Teale-Knapp
    tenotomy
    Terson
    Tessier
    Thomas
    three-snip punctum
    Tillett
    Toti
    Toti-Mosher
    Townley-Paton
    trabeculectomy
    Trainor
    Trainor-Nida
    transfixion of iris
    transplantation of ocular
      muscle
    Trantas
    trapdoor scleral buckle
    Tripier
    Troutman
    Truc
    Tudor Thomas
    tumbling technique cataract
      extraction
    Ulloa
    Van Milligen
    Veirs
    Verhoeff
    Verhoeff-Chandler
    Verwey
    Vogt

Additional Entries

operations *(continued)*
- Von Ammon
- von Blaskovics-Doyen
- Waldhauer
- Walter Reed
- Watzke
- Weeker
- Weeks
- Weisinger
- Wendell Hughes
- Werb
- West
- Weve
- Wharton-Jones
- Wheeler
- Wheeler-Reese
- Wicherkiewicz
- Wiener
- Wies
- Wilmer
- Wolfe
- Worst
- Worth
- Wright
- Young
- Z-plasty
- Ziegler
- Zylik

ophryon
Ophthaine
Ophthalas laser
Ophthalgan
ophthalmagra
ophthalmalgia
ophthalmatrophia
ophthalmectomy
ophthalmencephalon
ophthalmia
- actinic ray o.
- catarrhal o.
- caterpillar o.
- eczematosa, o.
- Egyptian o.
- flash o.
- gonorrheal o.
- granular o.
- jequirity o.
- metastatic o.
- scrofulous o.
- spring o.
- strumous o.
- sympathetic o.
- transferred o.
- ultraviolet ray o.
- varicose o.

ophthalmia neonatorum
ophthalmia nodosa
ophthalmiac
ophthalmiatrics
ophthalmic
ophthalmic arteries
ophthalmic cup
ophthalmic ganglion
ophthalmic migraine
ophthalmic nerve
ophthalmic plexus
ophthalmic reaction
ophthalmic solution
ophthalmic vein, inferior
ophthalmic vein, superior
ophthalmic video system
ophthalmitic
ophthalmitis
ophthalmoblennorrhea

Additional Entries

ophthalmocele
ophthalmocopia
ophthalmodesmitis
ophthalmodiaphanoscope
ophthalmodiastimeter
ophthalmodonesis
ophthalmodynamometer
ophthalmodynamometry
ophthalmodynia
ophthalmoeikonometer
ophthalmograph
ophthalmography
ophthalmogyric
ophthalmoleukoscope
ophthalmolith
ophthalmologic
ophthalmologist
ophthalmology
ophthalmomalacia
ophthalmomandibulomelic dysplasia
ophthalmomeningeal vein
ophthalmometer
ophthalmometroscope
ophthalmometry
ophthalmomycosis
ophthalmomyiasis
ophthalmomyitis
ophthalmomyositis
ophthalmomyotomy
ophthalmoneuritis
ophthalmoneuromyelitis
ophthalmopathy
    external o.
    internal o.
ophthalmophacometer
ophthalmophantom
ophthalmophlebotomy

ophthalmophthisis
ophthalmoplasty
ophthalmoplegia
    basal o.
    exophthalmic o.
    external o.
    fascicular o.
    infectious o.
    internal o.
    internuclear o.
    nuclear o.
    orbital o.
    Parinaud's o.
    total o.
    progressive o.
ophthalmoplegic
ophthalmoplegic migraine
ophthalmoptosis
ophthalmoreaction
    Calmette's o.
ophthalmorrhagia
ophthalmorrhea
ophthalmorrhexis
ophthalmoscope
    binocular o.
    direct o.
    ghost o.
    indirect o.
    Schepens binocular indirect o.
ophthalmoscopy
    direct o.
    indirect o.
    medical o.
    metric o.
    red free light o.
ophthalmostasis
ophthalmostat

Additional Entries

ophthalmostatometer
ophthalmosteresis
ophthalmosynchysis
ophthalmothermometer
ophthalmotomy
ophthalmotonometer
ophthalmotonometry
ophthalmotoxin
ophthalmotrope
ophthalmotropometer
ophthalmovascular
ophthalmovascular choke
ophthalmoxerosis
Ophthascan "S"
Ophthetic
Ophthochlor
Ophthocort
OPMI 6C-FC/XY operating microscope (Carl Zeiss)
opsin
opsiometer
opsoclonia
Optacryl
Optacryl contact lens
Optemp cautery
optesthesia
optic
optic angle
optic aphasia
optic atrophy, primary
optic atrophy, secondary
optic axis
optic canal
optic center
optic chiasm
optic cup
optic decussation
optic disk

optic foramen
optic evagination
optic foramen of sclera
optic foramen of sphenoid bone
optic hyperesthesia
optic iridectomy
optic keratoplasty
optic lemniscus
optic (II) nerve
optic neuritis
optic orbital ganglion
optic papilla
optic radiation
optic recess
optic stalk
optic sulcus
optic vesicle
optical
optical alexia
optical axis
optical density method
optical image
optical iridectomy
Optical Radiation intraocular lens
optici
optician
opticianry
opticist
Opti-Clean II
opticociliary
opticociliary neurectomy
opticocinerea
opticofacial winking reflex
opticokinetic
opticonasion
opticopupillary
Opticrom

Additional Entries

optics
opticum chiasma
Optikem International
optimeter
Optimyd
Optisoap
Opti-Soft Solution
optist
Opti-Tears drops
Opti-zyme
optoblast
optogram
optokinetic nystagmus
optomeninx
optometer
optometer reflexes
optometrist
optometry
optomotor reflexes
optomyometer
optophone
optotype
ora
    o. serrata retinae
Oratol
orb
orbicular
orbiculare
orbicularis oculi muscle
orbicularis reaction
orbicularis reflex
orbicularis sign
orbiculi
orbiculoanterocapsular fibers
orbiculus
    o. ciliaris
orbit
orbita

orbitae
orbital
orbital abscess
orbital aneurysm
orbital apex
orbital arch of frontal bone
orbital border of sphenoid bone
orbital canal
orbital canal, anterior internal
orbital canal, posterior internal
orbital cellulitis
orbital crest
orbital decompression
orbital fasciae
orbital fat pads
orbital floor
orbital hypertelorism
orbital hypotelorism
orbital implant
orbital margins
orbital opening
orbital ophthalmoplegia
orbital optic neuritis
orbital periosteum
orbital plane
orbital plane of frontal bone
orbital plate of ethmoid bone
orbital plate of frontal bone
orbital pseudotumor
orbital septum
orbital sulci of frontal bone
orbital wing of sphenoid bone
orbitale
orbitalis
orbitomalar foramen
orbitonasal
orbitonometer
orbitonometry

Additional Entries
_____
_____
_____
_____

orbitopathy
orbitostat
orbitotemporal
orbitotomy
organ
    accessory o's of eye
organum
    o. visus
orthofusor
Orthogon F bifocal lens
orthokeratology
orthometer
orthophoria
    asthenic o.
orthophoric
orthopia
orthopist
orthoposition
orthoptic
orthoptics
orthoptoscope
orthorater
orthoscope
orthoscopic
orthoscopy
orthropsia
os
    o. lacrimale
    o. orbiculare
    o. palatinum
    o. planum
    o. unguis
OS (oculus sinister - left eye)
oscillating vision
oscillopsia
Osmoglyn
osmotic
osteogenesis imperfecta
Ota's nevus
otolith apparatus
OU (oculi unitas - both eyes)
OU-180 ophthalmic chair &
    stand (Topcon Instrument)
Ovanite
overlap
over-refraction
overripe cataract
OWS (overwear syndrome)
Oxywet gas permeable contact
    lens

Additional Entries

Additional Entries

P

P & C (prism and cover test)
Pach-Pen hand-held pachymeter (Intermedics Intraocular)
Pach-Pen tonometer
pachyblepharon
pachyblepharosis
Pagenstecher operation
pain reaction
palatine bone
palinopsia
palpebra
    p. inferior
    p. superior
    p. tertius
palpebrae
palpebral fissure
palpebral fold
palpebral furrow
palpebral raphe
palpebral raphe, lateral
palpebralis
palpebrate
palpebration
palpebritis
palsy
PAN (periarteritis nodosa)
Panas operation
Pannu anterior chamber lens
pannus
    allergic p.
    degenerative p.
    phlyctenular p.
panophthalmia
panophthalmitis
panoptic

Panoptik bifocal lens
panoramic loupe
panretinal photocoagulation
pantankyloblepharon
pantoscope
    Keeler p.
pantoscopic
pantoscopic spectacles
pantoscopic tilt
Panum's fusion area
panuveitis
paper plate
papilla
    lacrimal p.
    optic p.
papillae
papillary stasis
papilledema
papillitis
    necrotizing p.
papillomacular bundle
papoculocerebrorenal dystrophy
parablepsia
paracentesis
    aqueous p.
paracentral scotoma
parachromatopsia
paradoxical diplopia
parafovea
parakinesis
parakinetic
parallax
    binocular p.
    crossed p.
    direct p.

Additional Entries

parallax *(continued)*
   heteronymous p.
   homonymous p.
   motion p.
   vertical p.
parallax test
paralysis
   abducens p.
   abducens-facial p.
   congenital abducens-
     facial p.
   congenital oculofacial p.
   conjugate p.
   internuclear p.
   ocular p.
   oculofacial p., congenital
paralytic ectropion
paralytic heterotropia
paralytic mydriasis
paralytic strabismus
paramacular
parasellar syndrome
parasympathetic
parasympatholytic
parasympathomimetic
Paredrine
Parel-Crock vitreous cutter
parenchymatous keratitis
paretic muscle
paries
   p. interior orbitae
   p. lateralis orbitae
   p. medialis orbitae
   p. superior orbitae
Parinaud's conjunctivitis
Parinaud's oculoglandular
   syndrome
Park speculum

Parke-Davis
Parker-Heath cautery
parophthalmia
parophthalmoncus
paropsis
Parrot's sign
pars
   p. caeca oculi
   p. caeca retinae
   p. ciliaris retinae
   p. iridica retinae
   p. lacrimalis musculi
     orbicularis oculi
   p. optica hypothalami
   p. optica retinae
   p. orbitalis glandulae
     lacrimalis
   p. orbitalis gyri frontalis
     inferioris
   p. orbitalis musculi
     orbicularis oculi
   p. orbitalis ossis frontalis
   p. palpebralis glandulae
     lacrimalis
   p. palpebralis musculi
     orbicularis oculi
   p. plana corporis ciliaris
pars plana approach
pars plana vitrectomy
pars planitis
pars plicata
partial cataract
PAS (peripheral anterior
   synechia)
Pascheff's conjunctivitis
passive illusion
PAT (prism adaptation test)
Patau's syndrome

Additional Entries

Paton knife
Paton spatula
pattern cut corneal graft
Paufique detached retina operation
Paufique keratoplasty
Paufique knife
Paufique synechiotomy
Paul retractor
Paxial pachymetry and/or axial length biometry (Biophysics, Medical)
PD (pupillary distance)
PDC-70 soft contact lens
PDR (proliferative diabetic retinopathy)
PE (pigment epithelium)
pearl cyst
pearls, Elschnig
pediculosis
    p. palpebrarum
Pel's crisis
pemphigoid
pemphigus
    ocular p.
pendular nystagmus
penetrating full thickness corneal graft
penetrating keratoplasty
Pentolair
PEO (progressive external ophthalmoplegia)
periarteritis nodosa
peribulbar
perichiasmal
periconchitis
pericorneal
pericorneal plexus

perifovea
perikeratic
perilenticular
Perimat 206
perimeter
    Allergan Humphrey p.
    Canon U.S.A. p.
    CILCO p.
    CooperVision Diagnostic Imaging p.
    Digilab p.
    Marco p.
    Topcon p.
perimetry
perinuclear cataract
periocular
periodic strabismus
periophthalmia
periophthalmic
periophthalmitis
perioptometry
periorbit
periorbita
periorbital
periorbititis
peripapillary
periphacitis
periphakitis
peripheral cataract
peripheral curve
peripheral iridectomy
peripheral vision
peripherophose
periphlebitis retinae
periretinal edema
periscopic
periscopic spectacles
peristriate

Additional Entries

peritarsal network
peritectomy
peritomist
peritomize
peritomy
perivasculitis
Perkins tonometer
Perlia's nucleus
Permaflex HGP
Permaflex-Thin
Permaflex-Thin 43
Permalens extended wear soft lenses
Permalens soft contact lens
Permalens-Aphakic
permeation analgesia
pernicious myopia
perosmic acid
PERRLA (pupils equal, round, reactive to light and accommodation)
pes
    p. corvinus
Peter operation
Petit's canal
petrificans conjunctivitis
petrolatum
PGC (pontine gaze center)
phacitis
phacoanaphylaxis
phacocele
phacocyst
phacocystectomy
phacocystitis
phacodonesis
phacoemulsification
phacoerysis
phacoglaucoma

phacohymenitis
phacoid
phacoiditis
phacoidoscope
phacolysis
phacolytic glaucoma
phacoma
phacomalacia
phacomatosis
phacometachoresis
phacometecesis
phacometer
phacopalingenesis
phacoplanesis
phacosclerosis
phacoscope
phacoscopy
phacoscotasmus
phacotoxic
phakic
phakogenic glaucoma
phakolytic glaucoma
phakomatoses
Pharmacia
Pharmacia Ophthalmics intraocular lens
Pharmaderm
Pharmafair
phenomenon
    Ascher's glass rod p.
    Bell's p.
    blood-influx p.
    Westphal-Piltz p.
phenylephrine hydrochloride
phenylketonuria
phi phenomenon
phlebophthalmotomy
phlyctena

Additional Entries

phlyctenar
phlyctenoid
phlyctenosis
phlyctenular conjunctivitis
phlyctenular keratitis
phlyctenular keratoconjunctivitis
phlyctenular pannus
phlyctenule
phlyctenulosis
PHM (posterior hyaloid membrane)
phoria
phoriascope
phorometer
phorometry
phoropter test
phoroscope
phorotone
phosphene
Phospholine Iodide
photerythrous
photesthesis
photic
photism
photochromic glasses
photochromic lens
photocoagulation
photocoagulator
    American Optical Company p.
    Mira p.
    Zeiss p.
photodysphoria
photoelectric vibration
photokeratoscope
    Allergan Medical Optics p.
    CooperVision Refractive Surgery p.

photometer
    Forster's p.
photone
photo-ophthalmia
    flash p.
photophobia
photophobic
photophthalmia
photopia
photopic
photopic adaptation
photopic vision
photopsia
photopsin
photopsy
photoptometer
photoptometry
photoreceptors
photoretinitis
PHPV (persistent hyperplasia of primary vitreous)
phthisis
    cornea, p.
    ocular p.
phycomycosis
    cerebral p.
physiologic blind spot
physiologic excavation
physiological astigmatism
physiological retina
physostigmine sulfate
PI (peripheral iridectomy)
pial sheath
Pick's vision
Pico operation
pigmentary glaucoma
pigmentary retinopathy
pigmented layer of ciliary body

Additional Entries

pigmented layer of eyeball
pigmented layer of iris
pigmented layer of retina
Pilocar
pilocarpine hydrochloride ophthalmic solution
pilocarpine nitrate ophthalmic solution
Pilocel
Pilokair
Pilopine HS
pimaricin
pimelopterygium
pinealoma
pinguecula
pinguicula
pinhole pupil
pink eye
pit
    Gaul's p's
    Herbert's p's
PKP (penetrating keratoplasty)
PKU (phenylketonuria)
Placido's disc
placode
    lens p.
plane
    Daubenton's p.
    eye-ear p.
    Frankfort horizontal p.
    Listing's p.
    orbital p.
    orbital p. of frontal bone
    regard, p. of
    visual p.
plano
planoconcave
planoconvex

Plano T lens
planum
    p. orbitale
plaque
    Hollenhorst p's
Plaquenil
plasmoid humor
plastic iritis
plastic lens
plate
    orbital p. of ethmoid bone
    orbital p. of frontal bone
    paper p.
    reticular p.
platycoria
platymorphic
platysmal reflex
pleoptics
plexiform layers
Plexiglas implant
plexus
    ophthalmic p.
    pericorneal p.
    stroma p., deep
Pliagel
plica
    p's ciliares
    p. lacrimalis
    p. palpebronasalis
    p. semilunaris conjunctivae
plombage
plus cyclophoria
PMMA (polymethylmethacrylate)
PN (periarteritis nodosa)
pneumococcus ulcer
pneumotonometer
p.o. (by mouth)

Additional Entries

pocket operation
POHS (presumed ocular histoplasmosis syndrome)
point
    cardinal p's
    conjugate p.
    convergence, p. of
    corresponding p's
    dispersion, p. of
    divergence, p. of
    eye p.
    far p.
    fixation p.
    focal p.
    lacrimal p.
    near p.
    near p., absolute
    near p., relative
    nodal p's
    regard, p. of
    supraorbital p.
poisoning degenerative cataract
polar cataract, anterior
polar cataract, posterior
polarized glasses
Polaroid vectograph slide
pole
    anterior p. of eyeball
    anterior p. of lens
    posterior p. of eyeball
    posterior p. of lens
poliosis
polus
    p. anterior bulbi oculi
    p. anterior lentis
Polyak operation
polyarteritis
Polycon

polycoria
    p. spuria
    p. vera
polyethylene sphere orbital implant
polymacon
polyopia
    binocular p.
    monophthalmica, p.
polyopsia
polyopy
Poly-Pred
Polysporin
Pompe's disease
pontine
Pontocaine
pore tip
porus
    p. opticus
position ametropia
positive accommodation
positive convergence
positive cyclophoria
positive eyepiece
positive vertical divergence
Posner-Schlossman syndrome
postchiasmatic eminence
posterior chamber
posterior discission
posterior embryotoxon
posterior lamina
posterior pole of eyeball
posterior pole of lens
posterior scleritis
posterior sclerotomy
posterior staphyloma
posterior symblepharon

Additional Entries

posterior synechia
posterior uveitis
postmarital amblyopia
postocular
postocular neuritis
postorbital
potassium hydroxide
Potter's syndrome
Poulard entropion
Poulard-Pochissov operation
Power's operation
PP (punctum proximum of convergence)
PPRF (paramedian pontine reticular formation)
PR (presbyopia)
Prader-Willi syndrome
prairie conjunctivitis
Precision Cosmet intraocular lens
Predair
Predair Forte
Predair-A
Predate
Pred Forte
Pred Mild
prednisolone sodium phosphate ophthalmic solution
Predsulfair
Preflex
Prefrin
Prefrin-A
prelacrimal
preliminary iridectomy
Prentice's rule
preparatory iridectomy
presbyopia
presbyopic
presbytia
presbytism
pressure
    intraocular p.
pressure dressing
pretectal nucleus
Prevost's sign
Preziosi operation
primary cataract
primary deviation
primary eye
primary glaucoma
primary persistent hyperplastic vitreous
primary vitreous
Prince clamp
Prince forceps
Prince rule
principal axis
principal foci
Priscoline
prism
    Maddox p.
    Risley's p.
    Wolff-Eisner p.
prism apex
prism ballast
prism bar
prism cover test
prism diopter
prismatic spectacles
prismoptometer
prismosphere
prisoptometer
p.r.n. (as needed)
PRO CEM-4 microscope
PRO-CMC 200 color video camera

Additional Entries

PRO CMC-300 Saticon camera
  (CooperVision Diagnostic
  Imaging)
Pro I 50/35/20 deg. camera
  (Kowa)
PRO/KOESTER WFSCM
  microscope
probe
    lacrimal p.
    Linde cryogenic p.
    Williams p.
    Worst p.
probing of lacrimonasal duct
process
    ciliary p's
    hamular p. of lacrimal bone
    uncinate p. of lacrimal
      bone
    zygomatico-orbital p. of
      maxilla
processus
    p. ciliares
    p. frontosphenoidalis ossis
      zygomatici
    p. zygomaticus maxillae
prodromal myopia
ProFree/GP weekly enzymatic
  cleaner (Allergan)
progressive cataract
progressive choroidal atrophy
progressive myopia
progressive ophthalmoplegia
progressive tapetochoroidal
  dystrophy
projecting staphyloma
projection
    erroneous p.
projection perimeter
projector
projectoscope
prolapse
    p. of the iris
prominence
    Ammon's scleral p.
proparacaine hydrochloride
  ophthalmic solution
proper substance of cornea
proper substance of sclera
Propine
Propper binocular indirect
  ophthalmoscope (Propper
  Mfg.)
Propper Manufacturing
Propper ophthalmoscope
proptometer
proptosis
prosthesis
    ocular p.
protanomaly
protanopia
protometer
provocative test
Prowazek's bodies
Prowazek-Greeff bodies
proximal convergence
PRP (panretinal
  photocoagulation)
PSC (posterior subcapsular
  cataract)
pseudoexfoliation
pseudoexophoria
pseudoexophthalmos
pseudo-Graefe's sign
pseudoisochromatic colors
pseudomembranous
  conjunctivitis

Additional Entries

_____
_____
_____
_____
_____

pseudomyopia
pseudonystagmus
pseudophakia
pseudoscopic vision
pseudostrabismus
pseudotumor
    orbital p.
pseudoxanthoma elasticum
PSP (progressive supranuclear palsy)
psychic blindness
pterygium
    congenital p.
    unguis, p.
PTG (Alcon applanation pneumatonograph)
ptosis
    adiposa, p.
    false p.
    Horner's p.
    lipomatosis, p.
    morning p.
    sympathica, p.
    waking p.
ptotic
puddler's cataract
Pulfrich phenomenon
pulpit spectacles
pulsating exophthalmos
puncta
punctate cataract
punctate retinitis
punctuate developmental cataract
punctum
punctumeter
pupil
    Adie's p.
    Argyll Robertson p.

pupil *(continued)*
    artificial p.
    Behr's p.
    bounding p.
    Bumke's p.
    cat's eye p.
    cornpicker's p.
    fixed p.
    Horner's p.
    Hutchinson's p.
    keyhole p.
    Marcus Gunn p.
    pinhole p.
    skew p's.
    stiff p.
    tonic p.
pupilla
pupillary
pupillary athetosis
pupillary axis
pupillary distance
pupillary margin of iris
pupillary membrane
pupillary reflex
pupillary paradoxic
pupillary zone
pupillatonia
pupillograph
pupillometer
pupillometry
pupilloplegia
pupilloscope
pupilloscopy
pupillostatometer
pupillotonia
pupil-to-root iridectomy
Purkinje's images
Purkinje-Sanson mirror images

Additional Entries

purpurogenous membrane
Purtscher's angiopathic
 retinopathy
Purtscher's disease
purulent conjunctivitis
purulent iritis
Putenney operation

P.V. Carpine
PXE (pseudoxanthoma
 elasticum)
pyophthalmia
pyophthalmitis
pyramidal cataract
Pyrex tube

Additional Entries

Additional Entries

Q

q. (every)
q.d. (every day)
q.i.d. (four times a day)
Q-switched YAG laser system
quadrant hemianopia
quadrantanopia
quadrantanopsia
quadrantic hemianopia
Quaglino's operation
Quevedo forceps
quinine amblyopia

Additional Entries

Additional Entries

R

radial keratotomy
radian
radiatio
    r. occipitothalamica (Gratioleti)
    r. optica
radiation
    occipitothalamic r.
    optic r.
radiation degenerative cataract
Radin-Rosenthal eye implant
radius
radiuscope
radiusgauge
radix
Raeder's syndrome
rainbow syndrome
rainbow vision
Ramsden's eyepiece
ramus
Randot test
R & R (recess-resect)
range
    r. of accommodation
raphe
    r., lateral palpebral
    r. palpebralis lateralis
    r. palpebrarum
    r. plica semilunaris
    r. posterior lamina
rasp
    Lundsgaard-Burch r.
Rathke's pouch tumor
Raverdino operation
ray
    convergent r.
Ray-Brunswick-Mack operation
Ray-McLean operaton
Raymond-Cestan syndrome
RD (retinal detachment)
reaction
    conjunctival r.
    hemiopic pupillary r.
    ophthalmic r.
    orbicularis r.
    pain r.
    vestibular pupillary r.
reading chart
real focus
reaper's keratitis
reattachment of retina
reattachment of choroid
receptor
    visual r.
recess
    optic r.
recession
    r. of ocular muscle
recessus
    r. opticus
Recklinghausen's disease
red blindness
red-green blindness
red reflex
Redmond Smith operation
reduced eye
reduplication cataract
Reese forceps

Additional Entries

Reese ptosis operation
Reese-Cleasby operation
Reese-Jones-Cooper operation
reflection
reflex
    accommodation r.
    attention r. of pupil
    audito-oculogyric r.
    blink r.
    chocked r.
    ciliary r.
    ciliospinal r.
    cochleopapillary r.
    conjunctival r.
    consensual r.
    consensual light r.
    convergency r.
    copper-wire r.
    corneal r.
    corneomandibular r.
    corneopterygoid r.
    corneomental r.
    crossed r.
    dazzle r.
    doll's eye r.
    emergency light r.
    eyeball compression r.
    eyeball-heart r.
    eyelid closure r.
    Gifford's r.
    Haab's r.
    iris contraction r.
    juvenile r.
    lacrimal r.
    lid r.
    light r.
    McCarthy's r.
    myopic r.

reflex *(continued)*
    oculocephalogyric r.
    oculopharyngeal r.
    oculopupillary r.
    oculosensory cell r.
    opticofacial winking r.
    orbicularis r.
    platysmal r.
    pupillary r.
    pupillary paradoxic r.
    paradoxic r.
    Ruggeri's r.
    shot-silk r.
    skin pupillary r.
    supraorbital r.
    tapetal light r.
    threat r.
    trigeminus r.
    water-silk r.
    Weiss's r.
    Westphal's pupillary r.
    Westphal-Piltz r.
reflex amaurosis
reflex amblyopia
reflex iridoplegia
refract
refracting media
refraction
    double r.
    dynamic r.
    ocular r.
    static r.
refractionist
refractive
refractive amblyopia
refractive ametropia
refractive error
refractivity

Additional Entries

refractometer
    Carl Zeiss r.
refractometry
refractor
    Allergan Humphrey r.
    Canon U.S.A. r.
    Coburn r.
    CooperVision Diagnostic
        Imaging r.
    Marco r.
    Reichert r.
    Topcon r.
Refresh
Refsum's disease
regio
    r. infraorbitalis
    r. orbitalis
region
    ciliary r.
    infraorbital r.
    ocular r.
    orbital r.
regular astigmatism
Reichert camera
Reichert Ful-Vue
    ophthalmoscope
Reichert Ful-Vue spot
    retinoscope
Reichert lensometer
Reichert MK IV binocular
    indirect ophthalmoscope
Reichert MK IV ophthalmoscope
Reichert Non-Contact II
    tonometer (NCT)
Reichert Ophthalmic Instruments
Reichert ophthalmodynamometer
Reichert radiusgauge
Reichert refractor
Reichert retinoscope
Reichert slit lamp
Reichert SR IV refractor
Reichert's membrane
Reis-Buckler's dystrophy
Reiter's syndrome
Rekoss disk
relative accommodation
relative hemianopia
relative hyperopia
relative strabismus
Relief
REM (rapid eye movements)
removal of foreign body from
    cornea
Remy separator
renal retinitis
repositor
        Nettleship iris r.
resection
rete mirabile
reticular keratitis
reticular plate
retina
retinal
retinal adaptation
retinal aplasia
retinal apoplexy
retinal asthenopia
retinal cone
retinal correspondence
retinal detachment
retinal embolism
retinal image
retinal isomerase
retinal migraine
retinal rivalry
retinal rods

Additional Entries

retinal staphyloma
retinascope
retinene isomerase
retinitis
    actinic r.
    apoplectic r.
    central angiospastic r.
    circinate r.
    Coat's r.
    diabetic r.
    exudative r.
    gravidarum, r.
    gravidic r.
    hypertensive r.
    Jacobson's r.
    Jensen's r.
    leukemic r.
    metastatic r.
    proliferating r.
    punctate r.
    renal r.
    serous r.
    solar r.
    splenic r.
    striate r.
    suppurative r.
    syphilitic r.
    uremic r.
retinitis pigmentosa
retinoblastoma
retinochoroid
retinochoroiditis
retinodialysis
retinograph
retinography
retinoid
retinol
retinomalacia

retinopapillitis
retinopathy
    bull's-eye r.
    central disk-shaped r.
    central serous r.
    circinate r.
    exudative r.
    leukemic r.
    pigmentary r.
    Purtscher's angiopathic r.
retinopexy
retinoschisis
retinoscope
    Keeler r.
    Reichert r.
retinoscopy
retinosis
retinotoxic
retraction syndrome
retractor
    Agrikola r.
    Arruga r.
    Ballen-Alexander r.
    Bronson-Turz r.
    Campbell r.
    Desmarres r.
    Goldstein lacrimal sac r.
    Harrison r.
    Jaeger r.
    Kirby r.
    Kronfeld r.
    Meller r.
    Paul r.
    Rizzuti iris r.
    Rollet r.
    Senn r.
    Stevenson r.
    Wilmer r.

Additional Entries

retrobulbar injection
retrobulbar neuritis
retrobulbar space
retro-illumination
retrolental
retrolental fibroplasia
retrolenticular
retro-ocular
retro-ocular space
retrotarsal
retrotarsal fold
Reuss' color chart
rhabdomyosarcoma
rhegmatogenous
ribbon-like keratitis
Riddoch phenomena
ridge
    supraorbital r.
Ridley anterior chamber lens implant
Ridley Mark II lens implant
Rieger's syndrome
Riesman's sign
Riley-Day syndrome
Riley-Smith syndrome
rima
    r. cornealis
    r. palpebrarum
ring
    Bonaccolto r.
    Caspar's r.
    ciliary r.
    ciliary r. of iris
    conjunctival r.
    glaucomatous r.
    greater r. of iris
    Kayser-Fleischer r.
    lenticular r.

ring *(continued)*
    lesser r. of iris
    Lowe's r.
    Maxwells's r.
    McKinney fixation r.
    Schwalbe's anterior border r.
    Schwalbe's r.
    Soemmering's r.
    Vossius r.
ring abscess
ring scotoma
ring ulcer
ringschwiele
Riolan's muscle
Ripault's sign
ripe cataract
Risley's prism
Ritter's fibers
rivalry
    binocular r.
    retinal r.
river blindness
rivus
    r. lacrimalis
Rizzuti iris retractor
RK (radial keratotomy)
RLF (retrolental fibroplasia)
RM-A6000 & RM-A6500 refractometers (Topcon Instrument)
RO 2002 photo slit lamp (Coburn Optical)
Robertson's sign
Rochat's test
Roche Laboratories
Rochon-Duvigneaud, bouquet of
rod
    retinal r's

Additional Entries

rod granule
rod vision
Rodenstock Combiline
 Instrument System (Coburn
 Optical)
Rodin orbital implant
Rolf dilator
roll
 scleral r.
roller forceps
Rollet retractor
Romana's sign
Ronne's nasal step
roof
 r. of orbit
root
 long r. of ciliary ganglion
 motor r. of ciliary ganglion
 oculomotor r. of ciliary
  ganglion
 sensory r. of ciliary
  ganglion
 short r. of ciliary ganglion
Roper-Hall localizer
Rosa-Berens orbital implant
rosacea keratitis
rose bengal
Rosenburg operation
Rosengren operation
Rosenmuller's body
Rosenmuller's gland
Ross Laboratories
rotary cutting tip
rotatory nystagmus
Roth-Bielschowsky syndrome
Roth's spots
Rothmund-Thomson syndrome
roto extraction
Rouget's muscle
Rovda operation
Rowbotham operation
Rowinski operation
RP (retinitis pigmentosa)
RPE (retinal pigment
 epithelium)
RT-1 refractor (Marco)
Rubbrecht operation
rubeosis iridis
Rubinstein cryoprobe
rudiment
 lens r.
Ruedemann operation
Ruedemann eye implant
ruffed canal
Ruggeri's reflex
Ruiz plano fundus lens implant
Ruysch's tunic
Rycroft operation

Additional Entries

S

S (spherical lens)
saburral amaurosis
sac
    lacrimal s.
saccade
saccadic
sacculus
    s. lacrimalis
saccus
    s. conjunctivae
Sachs' disease
Saemisch operation
Saenger's sign
Safar operation
sagittal axis of eye
sagittal axis of Fick
Salus sign
Salzmann's nodular corneal dystrophy
Sanders' operation
Sanders' disease
Sandhoff's disease
San Filippo disorder
sanguineous cataract
Sanson's images
Sappey's fibers
sarcomatosum
    s. senilis
    s. spasticum
    s. uveae
satellite lesion
Sato operation
Sato keratoconus
Sattler's layer
Sattler's veil

Sauflon 70 contact lens
Sauflon extended wear soft lens
Savin operation
saw
    Stryker s.
Sayoc operation
SBP-1000 automated perimeter (Topcon Instrument)
SBV (single binocular vision)
SC (without correction)
scaphoid
Scarpa's staphyloma
Schacher's ganglion
Scheie akinesia
Scheie classification
Scheie electrocautery
Scheie operation
Scheie technique
schematic eye
Schepens binocular indirect ophthalmoscope
Schepens operation
Schering Corporation
Schilder's disease
Schimek operation
Schiotz tonometer
Schirmer test
schisis
Schlemm's canal
Schmalz's operation
Schnyder's crystalline dystrophy
Schon's theory
Schwalbe's anterior border ring
Schwalbe's line
Schwalbe's spaces

Additional Entries

Schweigger forceps
Schweigger perimeter
scieropia
scimitar scotoma
scintillating scotoma
scirrhophthalmia
scissors
    Aebli corneal s.
    Barraquer s.
    Castroviejo s.
    DeWecker eye s.
    DeWecker-Pritikin s.
    Gill s.
    Guist s.
    Katzin s.
    Knapp iris s.
    Mattis s.
    Maunoir s.
    Mayo s.
    McClure s.
    McGuire s.
    McPherson-Vannas s.
    McReynolds s.
    Noyes s.
    Stevens s.
    Vannas s.
    Walker s.
    Walker-Apple s.
    Walker-Atkinson s.
    Werb s.
    Westcott s.
SCL (soft contact lens)
sclera
    blue s.
sclerae
scleral
scleral buckle
scleral canal
scleral depressor
scleral fistula operation
scleral framework
scleral furrow
scleral lens
scleral plugs
scleral roll
scleral shortening
scleral spur
scleral staphyloma
scleral sulcus
scleral trabeculae
scleratitis
sclercorneal sulcus
sclerectasia
sclerectasis
sclerectoiridectomy
sclerectoiridodialysis
sclerectome
sclerectomy
sclerectomy with punch (Holth operation)
sclerectomy with scissors (Lagrange operation)
sclerectomy with trephine (Elliot operation)
scleriritomy
scleritis
    annular s.
    anterior s.
    brawny s.
    posterior s.
sclerochoroiditis
    s. anterior
    s. posterior
scleroconjunctival
scleroconjunctivitis
sclerocornea

Additional Entries

sclerocornea
sclerocorneal
sclerocorneal junction
scleroderma
scleroiritis
sclerokeratitis
sclerokeratoiritis
sclerokeratosis
scleromalacia
scleronyxis
sclerophthalmia
scleroplasty
sclerosing keratitis
sclerostomy
sclerotica
scleroticectomy
scleroticochoroidal canal
scleroticochoroiditis
scleroticonyxis
scleroticopuncture
scleroticotomy
sclerotitis
sclerotome
sclerotomy
 anterior s.
 posterior s.
sclerotomy with drainage
sclerotomy with exploration
sclerotomy with removal of foreign body
Scobee hook
scopolamine
scoterythrous vision
scotodinia
scotoma
 absolute s.
 annular s.
 arc s.

scotoma *(continued)*
 arcuate s.
 aural s.
 Bjerrum's s.
 central s.
 centrocecal s.
 color s.
 comet s.
 eclipse s.
 flittering s.
 hemianoptic s.
 insular s.
 junction s.
 motile s.
 negative s.
 paracentral s.
 peripapillary s.
 peripheral s.
 physiologic s.
 positive s.
 relative s.
 ring s.
 scintillating s.
 Seidel's s.
 unilateral altitudinal s.
scotomagraph
scotomata
scotomatous
scotometer
 Bjerrum's s.
scotometry
scotomization
scotopia
scotopic
scotopic vision
scotopsin
scotoscopy
screen test

Additional Entries

scrofular conjunctivitis
scrofulous ophthalmia
scrofulus keratitis
Searcy trephine
sebaceous glands of conjunctiva
seborrheic blepharitis
second sight
secondary axis
secondary cataract
secondary deviation
secondary eye
secondary glaucoma
secondary keratitis
secondary vitreous
sector iridectomy
sedimentary cataract
Seeligmuller's sign
Seidel scotoma
Seidel sign
Selinger operation
sella turcica
semilunar fold
senile cataract
senile cortical degenerative
    cataract
senile disciform degeneration
senile ectropion
senile halo
senile macular exudative
    choroiditis
senile nuclear degenerative
    cataract
Senn retractor
sensory root of ciliary ganglion
SeptiSoak
septum
    orbital s.
Sereine

serous chorioretinopathy
serous iritis
serous retinitis
serpiginous keratitis
setting-sun sign
SFP (simultaneous foveal
    perception)
shadow test
Shaffer operation
shaft vision
Sharpoint
Sharpoint knife
Sharpoint microsurgical knife
    (Sharpoint)
Sharpoint slit knife (Sharpoint)
Sharpoint V-lance blade
    (Sharpoint)
Shearing lens
sheath
    arachnoid s.
    optic nerve, s. of
    pial s.
Sheets lens
Sheiner principle
shell implant
Sherrington's law
shield
    eye s.
    Mueller s.
shipyard conjunctivitis
shipyard disease
shipyard eye
shipyard keratoconjunctivitis
short root of ciliary ganglion
short sight
short-scale contrast
shot-silk reflex
shot-silk retina

Additional Entries

Shugrue operation
Sichel knife
Sichi movable implant
Sichi orbital implant
siderosis
- s. bulbi
- s. conjunctivae

sight
- day s.
- far s.
- long s.
- near s.
- night s.
- old s.
- second s.
- short s.

sign
- Ballet's s.
- Bard's s.
- Barre's s.
- Berger's s.
- Brickner's s.
- Cantelli's s.
- Collier's s.
- doll's eye s.
- Enroth's s.
- Gifford's s.
- Graefe's s.
- Knie's s.
- Kocher's s.
- Mann's s.
- Marcus Gunn's pupillary s.
- Munson's s.
- orbicularis s.
- Parrot's s.
- Prevost's s.
- pseudo-Graefe's s.
- Riesman's s.

sign *(continued)*
- Ripault's s.
- Robertson's s.
- Romana's s.
- Saenger's s.
- Seeligmuller's s.
- setting-sun s.
- Skeer's s.
- Stellwag's s.
- Stimson's s.
- Suker's s.
- swinging flashlight s.
- Tellais's s.
- Theimich's lip s.
- Weber's s.
- Wernicke's s.
- Widowitz's s.
- Wilder's s.
- Wood's s.

Silastic implant
silicone meshed motility orbital implant
siliculose cataract
siliquose cataract
Silisoft
sillonneur
Silva Costa operation
Silver-Hildreth eyelid operation
silver-wire reflex
Simcoe anterior chamber lens
Simcoe implant
Simcoe style handpiece
simple glaucoma
sinistrality
sinistrocularity
sinistrotorsion
Sinskey hook
Sinskey posterior chamber lens

Additional Entries

sinus
   s. circularis iridis
   s. of anterior chamber
   s. of Maier
   s. venosus
Siphunculina
   S. funicola
SITE LASAG microruptor
SITE LASAG Topaz Nd:YAG laser
SITE Microsurgical Systems
SITE-TXR Microsurgical System (SITE)
Sjogren's syndrome
Skeer's sign
skew deviation
skew pupil
skiametry
skiascope
skiascopy
skin pupillary reflex
slant muscle operation
slit beam of vertical light
slit lamp
slit lamp biomicroscope
SMD (senile macular degeneration)
Smart forceps
Smith eyelid operation
Smith Kline & French Laboratories
Smith knife
Smith orbital implant
Smith trabeculotomy
Smith-Fisher knife
Smith-Fisher spatula
SMP (simultaneous macular perception)
snare
   Banner s.
Snellen's chart
Snellen ptosis operation
Snellen vectis
Snellen's reform eye
Snellen's test
Snellen's test type
snow blindness
snow glasses
snowflake cataract
snowstorm cataract
SO (superior oblique)
Soaclens
Soakare
sodium fluorescein ophthalmic solution
sodium sulfacetamide ophthalmic ointment
sodium sulfacetamide ophthalmic solution
Soemmering's foramen
Soemmering's ring
Soemmering's ring cataract
Soemmering's spot
SOF (superior orbital fissure)
Sofact II soft contact lens
Sof-Form
Sof-Form II soft contact lens
Soflens
soft cataract
soft lens
Soft Mate
Soft Mate saline solution
Soft Mate soft contact lens
Soft Mate II soft contact lens
Soft Mate B soft contact lens
Soft Mate DW soft contact lens

Additional Entries

Soft Mate EW soft contact lens
Softcon
Softcon soft contact lens
Soft Therm
solar retinitis
solid silicone with Supramid mesh orbital implant
solid vision
SoluMedrol
solution
    antazoline phosphate ophthalmic s.
    atropine sulfate s.
    carbachol ophthalmic s.
    cyclopentolate hydrochloride s.
    demecarium bromide ophthalmic s.
    dexamethasone sodium s.
    epinephrine bitartrate ophthalmic s.
    homatropine hydrobromide ophthalmic s.
    hydroxyamphetamine s.
    hydrobromide ophthalmic s.
    idoxuridine ophthalmic s.
    isofuraphate s.
    ophthalmic s.
    neomycin sulfate, polymyxin B sulfate and gramicidin ophthalmic s.
    phenylephrine hydrochloride ophthalmic s.
    pilocarpine hydrochloride ophthalmic s.
    pilocarpine s.
    nitrate ophthalmic s.

solution *(continued)*
    prednisolone sodium phosphate ophthalmic s.
    proparacaine hydrochloride ophthalmic s.
    sodium fluorescein ophthalmic s.
    sodium sulfacetamide ophthalmic s.
    zinc sulfate ophthalmic s.
Sondermann's canal
Soquette soaking solution
Soria operation
Soriano operation
soul blindness
Sourdille keratoplasty
Sourdille ptosis operation
Sovereign bifocal lens
space
    circumlental s.
    Fontana's s's
    interlamellar s's
    intervaginal s's of optic nerve
    retrobulbar s.
    retro-ocular s.
Spaeth cystic bleb operation
Spaeth ptosis operation
spasm
    facial s.
    nictitating s.
    winking s.
spasmodic mydriasis
spasmodic strabismus
spasmus nutans
spastic ectropion
spastic entropion
spastic mydriasis

Additional Entries

spatium
　ss. anguli
　ss. anguli iridis (Fontanae)
spatula
　Green double s.
　Kirby iris s.
　Knapp s.
　Smith-Fisher s.
　Tooke s.
　Paton s.
SPC (simultaneous prism and cover) test
spear developmental cataract
Speas strabismus operation
spectacles
　compound s.
　decentered s.
　divided s.
　Masselon's s.
　mica s.
　pantoscopic s.
　periscopic s.
　prismatic s.
　pulpit s.
　stenopeic s.
　tinted s.
　wire frame s.
spectrocolorimeter
spectrum
　ocular s.
　visible s.
specular image
specular microscope
speculum
　Clark eye s.
　eye s.
　Guyton-Park lid s.
　Lancaster lid s.

speculum *(continued)*
　Park s.
　stop s.
Spencer-Watson operation
Spencer-Watson Z-plasty
sph. (spherical lens)
sphenoccipital fissure
sphenoidal fissure
sphenomaxillary fissure
sphenoorbital suture
sphenorbital
spherical
sphero-cylindrical
sphincter
　s. oculi
　s. of eye
　s. pupillae
sphincter muscle of pupil
sphincterectomy
sphincterolysis
sphingolipidoses
Spielmeyer-Vogt disease
spinal mydriasis
spindle
　Krukenberg s.
spindle cataract
spiral field
spiral of Tillaux
SPK (superficial punctate keratitis)
splenic retinitis
splitting of lacrimal papilla
spongy iritis
spoon
　Bunge s.
　Daviel s.
　Hess s.
　Kirby intracapsular lens s.

Additional Entries

spot
- acoustic s.
- Bitot's s.
- blind s.
- blue s.
- Brushfield's s.
- cherry-red s.
- cribriform s.
- eye s.
- Mariotte's s.
- Maxwell's s.
- Roth's s.
- Soemmering's s.
- Tay's s.
- yellow s.

spreading factor
spring conjunctivitis
spring ophthalmia
springing mydriasis
Spurway syndrome
squamous seborrheic blepharitis
Squid apparatus
squint angle
squint deviation
squirrel plague conjunctivitis
SR (superior rectus)
SR IV subjective refractor (Reichert)
SRNV (subretinal neovascularization)
SSPE (subactue sclerosing panencephalitis)
stalk
- optic s.

Stallard eyelid operation
Stallard flap operation
Stallard-Liegard suture
standard Project-O-Chart projector (Reichert)
staphyloma
- annular s.
- anterior s.
- ciliary s.
- corneal s.
- equatorial s.
- intercalary s.
- posterior s.
- projecting s.
- retinal s.
- scleral s.
- Scarpa's s.
- uveal s.

staphylomatous
star
- lens s's
- Winslow's s's

stare
Stargardt's disease
stasis
- papillary s.

static perimeters
static refraction
stationary cataract
steepest meridian
stella
- s. lentis hyaloidea
- s. lentis iridica

stellate cataract
Stellwag's sign
Stellwag's symptom
stenocoriasis
stenopeic
stenopeic disk
stenopeic iridectomy
stenopeic spectacles

Additional Entries

stenophotic
step graft, corneal
stereocampimeter
stereogram
stereo-ophthalmoscope
stereo-orthopter
stereophorometer
stereophoroscope
stereopsis
stereoscope
steroscopic vision
Steri-Units (Alcon)
Stevens scissors
Stevens-Johnson syndrome
Stevenson retractor
Stifel's figure
stiff pupil
stigmatometer
stigmatoscope
stigmatoscopy
Stiles-Crawford effect
stillicidium
    s. lacrimarum
Stilling's color test
Stilling-Turk-Duane syndrome
Still's disease
Stimson's sign
Stock operation
Stock-Spielmeyer-Vogt syndrome
Stocker operation
stop speculum
Stoxil
strabismic amblyopia
strabismic deviation
strabismus
    absolute s.
    accommodative s.

strabismus *(continued)*
    alternating s.
    bilateral s.
    binocular s.
    Braid's s.
    comitant s.
    concomitant s.
    constant s.
    convergent s.
    cyclic s.
    divergent s.
    dynamic s.
    external s.
    fixus s.
    horizontal s.
    incomitant s.
    intermittent s.
    internal s.
    kinetic s.
    latent s.
    manifest s.
    mechanical s.
    monocular s.
    monolateral s.
    muscular s.
    noncomitant s.
    nonconcomitant s.
    nonparalytic s.
    paralytic s.
    periodic s.
    relative s.
    spasmodic s.
    suppressed s.
    unilateral s.
    uniocular s.
    vertical s.
strabometer
strabometry

Additional Entries

strabotomy
Straith eyelid operation
Strampelli lens implant
Strampelli-Valvo operation
stratum
    cerebral s. of retina
    ganglionic s. of optic nerve
    ganglionic s. of retina
streak
    angioid s's
    Knapp's s's
streak retinoscopy
Streatfield operation
Streatfield-Fox operation
Streatfield-Snellen operation
stria
    ss. ciliares
striate keratitis
striate retinitis
stroboscopic disk
stroma
    s. of cornea
    s. of iris
    s., vitreous
stroma plexus
strumous ophthalmia
Stryker saw
Sturge-Weber syndrome
Sturm's conoid
Sturm's interval
stye
    meibomian s.
    zeisian s.
Style Keeper
Style Keeper contact lens
    carrying case (Allergan)
Suarez-Villafranca operation
subcapsular cataract

subchoroidal
subconjunctival
subconjunctival hemorrhage
subcortical alexia
subduct
subduction
sublatio
    s. retinae
subluxation of lens
subnormal accommodation
suborbital
subretinal
subscleral
substance
    cortical s. of lens
    exophthalmos-producing s.
    proper s. of cornea
    proper s. of sclera
substantia
    s. corticalis lentis
    s. lentis
    s. propria
    s. propria corneae
sugar-loaf cornea
Suker's sign
Sulamyd
sulcus
    chiasm, s. of
    infrapalpebral s.
    lacrimal s. of lacrimal bone
    lacrimal s. of maxilla
    optic s.
    orbital ss. of frontal bone
    scleral s.
    sclerocorneal s.
    orbitales lobi frontalis, s.
    supraorbital s.
Sulf-10

Additional Entries

sulfacetamide sodium
Sulfair
Sulfair 10
Sulfair 15
Sulfair Forte
sulfatide lipidosis
Sulphrin
Sulpred
Sulten-10
Summerskill operation
sunglasses
sunflower cataract
supercilia
superciliary
superciliary arch
supercilium
superficial punctate keratitis (SPK)
superimposition
superior arcade
superior fornix
superior oblique
superior orbital fissure
superior punctum
superior quadrantanopia
superior rectus
superior tarsus
superioris
superoccipital
supertraction conus
suppressed strabismus
suppurative choroiditis
suppurative keratitis
suppurative retinitis
suprachoroid
suprachoroid lamina
suprachoroidea
supraciliary
supraciliary canal
Supramid lens implant
supranuclear pathways
supraocular
supraoptic canal
supraoptic commissure
supraorbital
supraortibal arch of frontal bone
supraorbital artery
supraorbital canal
supraorbital foramen
supraorbital margin of orbit
supraorbital nerve
supraorbital neuralgia
supraorbital notch
supraorbital point
supraorbital reflex
supraorbital ridge
supraorbital sulcus
supraorbital vein
suprascleral
surface analgesia
Surgical Design
Surgidev intraocular lens
Surgikos
Surgiscope (Marco)
Surgisol
surplus field
sursumduction
sursumvergence
sursumversion
suspension
    cortisone acetate ophthalmic s.
    hydrocortisone acetate s. ophthalmic s.
suspensory ligament of lens

Additional Entries

sutura
   s. ethmoidomaxillaris
   s. frontolacrimalis
   s. infraorbitalis
   s. lacrimoconchalis
   s. lacrimomaxillaris
   s. sphenoorbitalis
sutural cataract
sutural developmental cataract
suture
   Custodis s.
   Davison-Geck s.
   Ethilon s.
   frontolacrimal s.
   Frost s.
   Gaillard-Arlt s.
   lacrimoconchal s.
   lacrimomaxillary s.
   lacrimoturbinal s.
   McLean s.
   sphenoorbital s.
   transverse s. of Krause
Swan syndrome
Swan incision
swimming pool conjunctivitis
swinging light test
swinging flashlight sign
Swiss blade breaker and holder
syllabic blindness
Sylvian syndrome
symblepharon
   anterior s.
   posterior s.
   total s.
symblepharopterygium
symmetric
sympathetic iridoplegia
sympathetic iritis

sympathetic nerve
sympathetic pathway
sympathetic ophthalmia
sympathetic uveitis
sympathizing eye
sympatholytic
sympathomimetic
symptom
   Berger's s.
   Haenel s.
   halo s.
   Liebreich's s.
   rainbow s.
   Stellwag's s.
   Wernicke's s.
symptomatic blepharospasm
synaphymenitis
syncanthus
synchysis
   s. scintillans
syndrome
   accommodative effort s.
   Adie's s.
   adherence s.
   Alport's s.
   Angelucci's s.
   Anton's s.
   Apert's s.
   Ascher's glass rod s.
   Axenfeld's s.
   Balint's s.
   Bassen-Kornzweig s.
   Batten-Mayou s.
   Benedikt's s.
   Bielschowsky-Lutz-Cogan s.
   Bloch-Stauffer s.
   Bloch-Sulzberger s.
   Bonnier's s.

Additional Entries

syndrome *(continued)*
    Brown's s.
    Brushfield-Wyatt s.
    cat's eye s.
    Cestan-Chenais s.
    Chandler's s.
    Charlin's s.
    chiasma s.
    chiasmatic s.
    co-contraction s.
    Cogan's s.
    Crouzon's s.
    Duane's s.
    Forssman's carotid s.
    Foville's s.
    Francois' s.
    Gunn's s.
    Hallermann-Streiff s.
    Hallermann-Streiff-Francois s.
    Harada's s.
    Heidenhaim's s.
    hereditary benign intraepithelial s.
    Homen's s.
    Horner's s.
    Horner-Bernard s.
    Hunter's s.
    Hunter-Hurler s.
    Hurler's s.
    hyperophthalmopathic s.
    jaw-winking s.
    Johnson s.
    Kennedy's s.
    Kiloh-Nevin s.
    Lawford's s.
    Lowe's s.
    Lowe-Terry-Machlachan s.

syndrome *(continued)*
    Marcus Gunn's s.
    Melkerssons's s.
    Melkersson-Rosenthal s.
    Millard-Gubler s.
    Mobius' s.
    Monakow's s.
    Parinaud's s.
    oculoglandular s.
    Potter's s.
    Prader-Willi s.
    Raymond-Cestan s.
    Rieger's s.
    Riley-Smith s.
    Rothmund-Thomson s.
    Sjogren's s.
    Spurway s.
    Stevens-Johnson s.
    Stilling-Turk-Duane s.
    tegmental s.
    Treacher-Collins s.
    Vogt-Koyanagi s.
    Waardenburg's s.
    Waardenburg's-Klein s.
synechia
    annular s.
    anterior s.
    circular s.
    posterior s.
    total anterior s.
    total posterior s.
synechiae
synechotome
synechotomy
synephris
syneresis
synergist

Additional Entries

synizesis
    s. pupillae
synkinesis
synkinetic
synophthalmia
synophthalmus
synoptophore

synoptophore test
synoptoscope
Synsoft bifocal soft contact lens
syphilitic retinitis
Szymanowski operation
Szymanowski-Kuhnt operation

Additional Entries

Additional Entries

T

305 monocular indirect ophthalmoscope (Reichert)
taco test
Taillefer's valve
Takahashi forceps
Takayasu's disease
tamponage
tangent screen
Tangier disease
Tansley operation
TAP (tension applanation)
tapetal light reflex
tapetochoroidal dystrophy
tapetoretinopathy
tapetum
    t. lucidum
    t. oculi
tarsal arteries, lateral
tarsal arteries, medial
tarsal canal
tarsal gland
tarsal muscle
tarsal plate
tarsocheiloplasty
tarsomalacia
tarso-orbital
tarsoplasia
tarsoplasty
tarsorrhaphy
tarsotomy
tarsus
    t. inferior palpebrae
    t. superior palpebrae
Tasia operation
tattooing
    t. of the cornea
Tay's choroiditis
Tay's spot
Tay-Sachs disease
Teale-Knapp operation
tear duct
tear gas
Tearfair
Tearisol
tears
    crocodile t.
Tears Naturale
Tears Plus
Tears Renewed
tectonic keratoplasty
tefilcon
Teflon orbital floor orbital implant
tegmental syndrome
tela
    t. cellulosa
    t. conjunctiva
telebinocular
telecanthus
Telfa dressing
Telfa plastic film dressing
Tellais's sign
temporal arteriole of retina, inferior
temporal arteriole of retina, superior
temporal arteritis
temporal crescent

Additional Entries

temporal hemianopia
temporal retina
temporal venule of retina,
   inferior
temporal venule of retina,
   superior
tenectomy
Tennant lens
tenonitis
Tenon's capsule
Tenon's fascia
Tenon's membrane
Tenon's space
tenotomize
tenotomy
   curb t.
tenotomy of ocular tendon
Tensilon
tension
   intraocular t.
Terrien's ulcer
Terry keratometer (TK)
Terson operation
tertiary vitreous
tessellated fundus
test
   alternate cover t.
   Amsler grid t.
   applanation tonometry t.
   Berman locator t.
   binocular indirect
      ophthalmoscope t.
   cheiroscope t.
   color vision t.
   corneal staining t.
   cover t.
   Cuignet's t.
   darkroom t.

test *(continued)*
   Duane's t.
   Dvorine t.
   echo-ophthalmography t.
   Ehrmann's t.
   electroretinography t.
   exophthalmometry t.
   fluorescein angiography t.
   gonioscopy t.
   Graefe's t.
   Hering's t.
   Holmgren t.
   Ishihara color t.
   Jenning's t.
   Klein keratoscope t.
   lantern t.
   light and color perception t.
   Maddox rod t.
   Nagel's t.
   ophthalmodynamometry t.
   ophthalmoscopy direct t.
   ophthalmoscopy indirect t.
   ophthalmoscopy red free
      light t.
   parallax t.
   phoropter t.
   provocative t.
   Schiotz tonometry t.
   Schirmer t.
   screen test t.
   shadow t.
   slit lamp t.
   Snellen's t.
   Stilling's color t.
   synoptophore t.
   tonography t.
   transillumination t.
   visual field t.

Additional Entries

test *(continued)*
   water provocative t.
   Welland's t.
   Wilbrand's t.
test type
   Jaeger's t.
   Snellen's t.
tetartanopia
tetartanopic
tetartanopsia
tetracaine hydrochloride
tetrachromic
tetrahydrozoline hydrochloride ophthalmic solution
tetranopsia
tetrastichiasis
text blindness
thalamolenticular
Theimich's lip sign
thelaziasis
theory
   Hering's t.
   Schon's t.
   Young-Helmholtz t.
therapeutic iridectomy
thimerosal
Thomas cryoptor
Thomas operation
Thomson syndrome
Thorpe forceps
threat reflex
three-mirror contact lens
three-snip punctum
threshold
   achromatic t.
Thygeson's keratitis
thyrotoxic exophthalmos
thyrotropic exophthalmos

tic
   local t.
   motor t.
t.i.d. (three times a day)
tie-over dressing
tigroid fundus
tigroid retina
Tillett operation
Tillyer bifocal lens
timolol maleate
Timoptic
tinted spectacles
tissue
   Kuhnt's intermediary t.
Titan
Titan II cleaning solution
Titan liquid cleaner
Titmus bifocal lens
Titmus glaretester
Titmus Optical
Titmus test
TK (Terry keratometer)
TN (tension)
TNO stereo test
tobacco amblyopia
tobramycin
Tobrex
Todd cautery
tolazoline
Tolentino vitreous cutter
Tolosa-Hunt syndrome
tonic pupil
tonogram
tonograph
tonography
tonometer
   air-puff t.
   applanation t.

Additional Entries

tonometer *(continued)*
    Goldmann's applanation t.
    impression t.
    indentation t.
    MacKay-Marg electronic t.
    McLean t.
    pneumatic t.
    Schiotz t.
tonometry
    applanation t.
    digital t.
    indentation t.
Tono-Pen tonometer (Intermedics Intraocular)
Tooke knife
Tooke spatula
Topcon aspheric lens
Topcon camera
Topcon chart projector
Topcon Instrument Corporation of America
Topcon lensometer
Topcon perimeter
Topcon refractor
Topcon refractometer
Topcon SL-2E slit lamp
Topcon SL-3E slit lamp
Topcon SL-6E slit lamp
Topcon VT-SE vision tester
Topcon VT-D5 vision tester
topical anesthesia
toric lens
Torisoft soft contact lens
torsion
torsional diplopia
torticollis
Total
total anterior synechia
total blindness
total cataract
total hyperopia
total posterior synechia
total symblepharon
Toti operation
Toti-Mosher operation
Townley-Paton operation
toxic amblyopia
toxic cataract
toxoplasmosis
TPI (treponema pallidum immobilization)
trabecular meshwork
trabeculectomy
trabeculotomy
trachoma
    Arlt's t.
trachoma body
trachoma gland
trachomatous conjunctivitis
trachomatous keratitis
tract
    uveal t.
Trainor-Nida operation
transferred ophthalmia
transfixion of iris
transformer, wall mounted (Propper Mfg.)
transillumination test
transition zone
transocular
transplantation of ocular muscle
transposition
transverse suture of Krause
Trantas operation
Trantas dots
trap door technique

Additional Entries

traumatic amblyopia
traumatic cataract
traumatic degenerative
   cataract
traumatic glaucoma
Treacher-Collins syndrome
tremulous cataract
tremulous iris
trephine
   Brown-Pusey t.
   Dimitry t.
   Elliott corneal t.
   Gradle t.
   Grieshaber t.
   Lichtenberg t.
   Mueller t.
   Searcy t.
Tresoft
Tresoft soft contact lens
Tretherm
triad
   Charcot's t.
trial case
trial frame
triangle
   frontal t.
   Wernicke's t.
trichiasis
Trichothecium
   T. roseum
trichromat
trichromatic
trichromatism
trichromatopsia
trichromic
trifluorothymidine
trifocal glasses
trigeminal (V) nerve

trigeminus reflex
Tripier operation
triple vision
triplopia
tristichia
tritanomaly
tritanopia
tritanopic
tritanopsia
trochlea
   t. musculi obliqui
     superioris bulbi
   t. musculi obliqui
     superioris oculi
   t. of superior oblique
     muscle
trochlear fovea
trochlear (IV) nerve
troland
Troncosco tubular gonioscopic
   lens implant
trophic keratitis
tropia
Tropicacyl
tropicamide
troposcope
Troutman implant
Troutman operation
Truc flap
Truc operation
true hemianopia
tube
   Bowman's t.
   corneal t.
   fusion t.
   Jones Pyrex t.
tuber
   frontal t.

Additional Entries

tubercle
    lateral orbital t.
    lateral palpebral t.
Tudor Thomas graft
tularemic conjunctivitis
tularensis conjunctivitis
tumbling procedure
tunic
    fibrous t. of eyeball
    Ruysch's t.
tunica
    t. adnata oculi
    t. conjunctiva
    t. conjunctiva bulbi
    t. conjunctiva bulbi oculi
    t. conjunctiva palpebrarum
    t. fibrosa bulbi
    t. fibrosa oculi
    t. nervea of Brucke
    t. nervosa oculi
    t. ruyschiana
    t. vascularis oculi

tunica *(continued)*
    t. vasculosa bulbi
    t. vasculosa lentis
    t. vasculosa oculi
tunnel vision
Turner's syndrome
tutamen
    t. oculi
tutamina
    t. oculi
TVA (true visual acuity) Test System (Innomed)
twilight blindness
twilight vision
twin cone
tylosis
    t. ciliaris
tylotic
Tyndall effect
typhlology
typhlosis
typical coloboma
Tyrrell iris book

Additional Entries

U

ulcer
    annular u.
    catarrhal corneal u.
    pneumococcus u.
    ring u.
    serpiginous corneal u.
ulcus
    u. serpens corneae
Ulloa operation
Ultex lens implants
Ultramatic Project-O-Chart projector (Reichert)
Ultramatic Rx master phoroptor (Reichert)
Ultrascan Digital B system IV
ultraviolet ray ophthalmia
Ultex bifocal lens
umbrella iris
uncinate process of lacrimal bone
unguentum
    u. epinephrinae bitartratis ophthalmicum
unilateral altitudinal scotoma
unilateral hemianopia
unilateral strabismus
uniocular
uniocular hemianopia
uniocular strabismus
Unisol
Unisol 4
Universal conformer set
up-gaze
UPOC (Ultramatic Project-O-Chart projector)
upper hemianopia
upper retina
uratic conjunctivitis
uremic amaurosis
uremic amblyopia
uremic retinitis
Uribe orbital implant
Usher's syndrome
UV Nova Curve
uvea
uveal framework
uveal staphyloma
uveal tract
uveitis

Additional Entries

Additional Entries

V

V slit lamp (Marco)
VA (visual acuity)
VA magnetic orbital implant
valve
    Beraud's v.
    Bianchi's v.
    Bochdalek's v.
    Foltz's v.
    Hasner's v.
    Huschke's v.
    Taillefer's v.
van de Hoeve's disease
Van Iderstine Designs
Van Lint akinesia
Van Lint and Atkinson lid
    akinetic block
Van Lint injection
Van Milligen eyelid repair
    technique
vanadiumism
Vannas scissors
varicose ophthalmia
varicula
Varigray lens implant
Varilux lens implant
vas
    vv. sanguinea retinae
vascular circle of optic nerve
vascular funnel
vascular keratitis
Vasocidin
Vasoclear
Vasoclear A
Vasocon
Vasocon-A
Vasosulf
VE (visual efficiency)
VECP (visual evoked cortical
    potential)
vectograph
vein
    aqueous v's
    central v. of retina
    choroid v.
    conjunctival v's
    Kuhnt's postcentral v.
    lacrimal v.
    ophthalmic v., inferior
    ophthalmic v., superior
    ophthalmomeningeal v.
    supraorbital v.
Veirs operation
Veirs rod
velonoskiascopy
venae
    angularis, v.
    centralis retinae, v.
    choroidea, v.
    choroidea oculi, v.
    ciliares, v's
    ciliares anteriores, v's
    ciliares posteriores, v's
    conjunctivales, v's
    conjunctivales anteriores,
        v's
    conjunctivales posteriores,
        v's
    episclerales, v's
    facialis, v.
    facialis anterior, v.

Additional Entries

venae *(continued)*
    facialis communis, v.
    facialis posterior, v.
    lacrimalis, v.
    nasofrontalis, v.
    ophthalmic v., inferior
    ophthalmic v., superior
    ophthalmomeningea, v.
    palpebrales, v's
    palpebrales v's, inferiores
    palpebrales v's, superiores
    supraorbitalis, v.
    supratrochleares, v's
    vorticosae, v's
venter
    v. frontalis musculi occipitofrontalis
venula
    v. macularis superior
    v. medialis retinae
    v. nasalis retinae inferior
    v. nasalis retinae superior
    v. retinae medialis
    v. temporalis retinae inferior
    v. temporalis retinae superior
venulae
venule
    macular v., inferior
    macular v., superior
    medial v. of retina
    nasal v. of retina, inferior
    nasal v. of retina, superior
    temporal v. of retina, inferior
    temporal v. of retina, superior

VER (visual evoked response)
Verga's lacrimal groove
vergence
Verhoeff operation
Verhoeff forceps
Verhoeff-Chandler capsulotomy
vernal conjunctivitis
vernier acuity
vertex
    v. of cornea
vertical axis of eye
vertical diplopia
vertical hemianopia
vertical parallax
vertical phoria
vertical strabismus
Verwey operation
Verwey eyelid operation
vesicle
    lens v.
    ocular v.
    optic v.
vesicula
    v. ophthalmica
vesicular keratitis
vestibular nystagmus
vestibular pupillary reaction
vestibulo-ocular reflex
V-G slit lamp (Marco)
vibration
    photoelectric v.
vidarabine
Vieth-Mueller horopter
vifilcon A
Villasenor ultrasonic pachymeter (CILCO)
violet vision
Vira-A

Additional Entries

viral conjunctivitis
viral keratoconjunctivitis
Viroptic
virtual focus
Visalens
Visalens soaking/cleaning solution
VISC instrument
Viscoat viscoelastic material
visible spectrum
Visine
Visine A.C.
vision
    achromatic v.
    binocular v.
    central v.
    chromatic v.
    color v.
    day v.
    dichromatic v.
    direct v.
    double v.
    facial v.
    false v.
    finger v.
    foveal v.
    half v.
    halo v.
    haploscopic v.
    indirect v.
    iridescent v.
    monocular v.
    multiple v.
    night v.
    oscillating v.
    peripheral v.
    photopic v.
    Pick's v.
vision *(continued)*
    pseudoscopic v.
    rainbow v.
    rod v.
    scoterythrous v.
    scotopic v.
    shaft v.
    solid v.
    stereoscopic v.
    triple v.
    tunnel v.
    twilight v.
    violet v.
    word v.
Vistakon
Vistamarc
Vistamaster Giantscope (Reichert)
visual
visual acuity
visual agnosia
visual angle
visual axis
visual cone
visual efficiency
visual evoked response
visual field
visual image
visual line
visual organ
visual plane
visual receptor
visualization
visualize
Visulas Nd:YAG laser (Carl Zeiss)
visuoauditory
visuognosis

Additional Entries

visuometer
visuopsychic
visuosensory
visuscope
vitelliform degeneration of Best
vitelliform macular
　degeneration
vitrectomy
vitreocapsulitis
vitreous
　　detached v.
　　primary v.
　　primary persistent
　　　hyperplastic v.
　　secondary v.
　　tertiary v.
vitreous body
vitreous bulge
vitreous chamber
vitreous detachment
vitreous face
vitreous floater
vitreous humor
vitreous membrane
vitreous opacity
vitreous stroma
vitreous-block glaucoma
vitreum
vitrina
　　v. ocularis
　　v. oculi
Vitrophage-Peyman Unit
　(CILCO)
V-lance blade (Sharpoint)
VOD (vision, right eye)
Vogt cataract

Vogt operation
Vogt-Koyanagi syndrome
Vogt-Koyanagi-Harada
　syndrome
Vogt-Spielmeyer disease
Volk conoid lens implant
Von Ammon operation
von Blaskovics-Doyen operation
von Gierke's disease
von Graefe cataract knife
　(Graefe)
von Graefe cystotome (Graefe)
von Graefe iris forceps (Graefe)
von Graefe knife needle
　(Graefe)
von Graefe muscle hooks
　(Graefe)
von Graefe sign
von Graefe syndrome
von Hippel operation
von Hippel's disease
von Hippel-Lindau disease
von Monakow's fibers
von Recklinghausen disease
von Willebrandt's knee
VOR (vestibulo-ocular reflex)
vortex
　　v. dystrophy
　　v. lentis
　　v. veins
VOS (vision, left eye)
Vossius' lenticular ring
V-pattern
VT-SE vision tester (Topcon
　Instrument)
vuerometer

Additional Entries

W

Waardenburg's syndrome
Waardenburg-Klein syndrome
Wachendorf's membrane
waking ptosis
Waldeyer's glands
Waldhauer operation
Walker Pharmacal
Walker scissors
Walker-Apple scissors
Walker-Atkinson scissors
Wallach LL100 (Wallach Surgical)
Wallach Mini Freezer (Wallach Surgical)
Wallach Surgical Devices
Wallach WA1000A (Wallach Surgical)
Wallach WA1000AB (Wallach Surgical)
Wallenberg syndrome
walleye
Walter Reed implant
wash
    eye w.
watch glass
water provocative test
watered-silk retina
water-silk reflex
Watzke operation
Weber's sign
Weck sponges
Weeker operation
Weeks operation
Weeks bacillus
Weill-Marchesani syndrome

Weisinger operation
Weiss's reflex
Welch 4-drop
welder's conjunctivitis
Welland's test
Werb scissors
Werb's operation
Werner's syndrome
Wernicke's encephalopathy
Wernicke's sign
Wernicke's symptom
Wernicke's triangle
Wesley Jessen lens
West operation
Westcott scissors
Westphal's pupillary reflex
Westphal-Piltz reflex
Wet-cote
wet dressing
Wet-N-Soak
wetting solution
Wharton-Jones (V-Y) operation
Wheeler knife
Wheeler operation
Wheeler-Reese operation
white cells
whorl
    lens w.
Wicherkiewicz eyelid operation
wide-angle glaucoma
widefield eyepiece
Widmark's conjunctivitis
Widowitz's sign
Wieger's ligament
Wiener operation

Additional Entries

Wies operation
Wilbrand's prism test
Wild operating microscope
Wilder cystotome
Wilder dilator
Wilder's sign
Wildgen-Reck localizer
Williams probes
Wilmer operation
Wilmer retractor
Wilson's degeneration
wing
    orbital w. of sphenoid bone
wing cell
winking
    jaw w.
Winslow's stars
wire frame spectacles
Wirt stereopsis test
Wirt test
Wolfe forceps
Wolfe operation
Wolfe's graft
Wolff ptosis operation
Wolff-Eisner test
Wolfring's glands
Wood's sign
word blindness
word vision
Worst probe
Worth forceps
Worth four-dot test (W4D)
Worth ptosis operation
Wrattan #47 filter
Wright operation
Wundt-Lamansky law
Wyeth Laboratories

Additional Entries

Wies' operation

X

xanthelasma
    generalized x.
xanthelasmatosis
xanthoma
    x. palpebrarum
    x. planum
xanthomatosis
    x. bulbi
    x. iridis
xanthomatous
xanthophane
xanthopsia
X-cel bifocal lens
xenophthalmia
xeroderma
    x. of Kaposi
    x. pigmentosum

xerodermatic
xerodermia
xeroma
xerophthalmia
xerophthalmus
xerosis
    x. conjunctival
    x. corneal
xerotic keratitis
X-Flo I/A machine
X-Pak I/A surgical system
X-Tender tubing set
X-Vee surgical system
XT (exotropia)
X(T) (intermittent exotropia)
Xylocaine

Additional Entries

Additional Entries

Y

YAG lasers
    Biophysic Medical y.
    Carl Zeiss y.
    CILCO y.
    Coherent Medical y.
    CooperVision Laser y.
    SITE y.

yellow mercuric oxide 1%
yellow mercuric oxide 2%
yellow spot
yoked muscles
Young operation
Young-Helmholtz
Y sutures

Additional Entries

Additional Entries

Z

zeisian gland
zeisian stye
Zeiss aspheric lens (Carl Zeiss)
Zeiss fundus camera
Zeiss fundus camera FF4
Zeiss Fundus Flash II Unit
Zeiss operating microscope
Zeiss photo slit lamp
Zeiss photocoagulator
Ziegler dilator
Ziegler knife
Ziegler knife needle
Ziegler operation
zinc sulfate ophthalmic solution
Zincfrin
Zinn's corona
Zinn's membrane
Z marginal tenotomy
Zollner's lines
Zolyse
zona
    z. ciliaris
    z. ophthalmica
zone
    ciliary z.
    extravisual z.
    interpalpebral z.
    pupillary z.
    transition z.

zone *(continued)*
    Zinn, z. of
zonula
    z. ciliaris
zonulae
zonular
zonular band
zonular cataract
zonular fibers
zonular keratitis
zonule
    ciliary z.
    lens z.
zonulitis
zonulolysis
zonulotomy
zonulysis
Z-plasty
zygoma
zygomatic foramen, interior
zygomatic foramen of Arnold, internal
zygomatic foramen, orbital
zygomatic foramen, posterior
zygomatico-orbital
zygomatico-orbital artery
zygomatico-orbital foramen
zygomatico-orbital process of maxilla
Zylik operation

Additional Entries

N. GUNN